Dr. Kathy's Health & Weight Loss Guide

The Whole Truth about Habits and Health
What Do We Eat?
Eating on the Go
Overweight? How to Lose It!

By

Dr. Kathy James

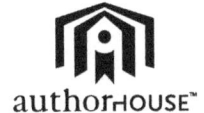

authorHOUSE™

1663 LIBERTY DRIVE, SUITE 200
BLOOMINGTON, INDIANA 47403
(800) 839-8640
WWW.AUTHORHOUSE.COM

This book is a work of non-fiction. Unless otherwise noted, the author and the publisher make no explicit guarantees as to the accuracy of the information contained in this book and in some cases, names of people and places have been altered to protect their privacy.

© 2005 Dr. Kathy James. All Rights Reserved.

No part of this book may be reproduced, stored in a retrieval system, or transmitted by any means without the written permission of the author.

First published by AuthorHouse 04/19/05

ISBN: 1-4208-1247-5 (sc)
ISBN: 1-4208-1248-3 (dj)

Library of Congress Control Number: 2004098779

Printed in the United States of America
Bloomington, Indiana

This book is printed on acid-free paper.

TABLE OF CONTENTS

PREFACE vii

ACKNOWLEDGMENTS ix

INTRODUCTION xi

PART ONE THE WHOLE TRUTH ABOUT HABITS AND HEALTH . 1
    Chapter One Bull's-eye: Target Health 3
    Chapter Two Habitually Healthy 10

PART TWO WHAT DO WE EAT? 19
    Chapter Three Food Choices: What and How Much? ... 21
    Chapter Four Nutrient Basics: Protein, Carbohydrates, and Fats 35
    Chapter Five Green Tips 49
    Chapter Six On the Go 57
    Chapter Seven Beat It! 63
    Chapter Eight Fiberlicious 69

PART THREE EATING ON THE GO 73
    Chapter Nine Planning Meals in Stride 75
    Chapter Ten Fabulous and Healthy Recipes 83

PART FOUR OVERWEIGHT? HOW TO LOSE IT! 99
    Chapter Eleven Ten Steps to Successful Weight Loss .. 101

APPENDIX A WEB RESOURCES 113

APPENDIX B HELPFUL WORKSHEETS (MAY BE COPIED) 115

GROCERY LIST 116

Growth Charts	118
TARGET HABIT WORKSHEET	**120**
Food Guide Pyramid	121
APPENDIX C NEW LABEL TERMINOLOGY	**122**
APPENDIX D SELECTED REFERENCES	**124**
INDEX	**126**

PREFACE

We are all busier than ever, and yet we are fatter than ever. We know more than ever before about what it takes to be healthy, but we're not. Working long hours and with hectic schedules, we have little extra time for family meals . . . let alone healthy ones. This is a practical book for busy people who don't have time to read a variety of nutrition books in order to obtain key health and nutritional information. This book is an easy reference that allows you to do a quick check of your current habits and food choices and then gives you the bottom line of what you need to know to make healthy food choices. The content is based on over 20 years of behavioral and nutritional counseling with families. Common questions and concerns make up the chapters of this book. The information is based on scientific information without extensive explanations. I gleaned it and simplified it for you!!

Whether it is a guide to how much protein family members need, how much sugar is in your cereal, how to have healthy bones, how to make healthy meals in a short period of time, eating out, or how to lose weight, you will find simple, direct answers within the chapters of this book. I include easy-to-read charts, bullet key information, and provide actual family experiences in sections called Family Time. Families often know what they're doing that's contributing to their being out of shape or to their medical problems, but they aren't certain where to start to correct the problem. I offer simple solutions for my patients while empowering you to achieve the desired healthy results. Each chapter ends with chapter highlights.

ACKNOWLEDGMENTS

Thank you to my husband who has always supported and believed in me through fat and thin!

To my many friends who offered their editorial services and encouragement—especially Stu, Dr. Pratt, Dr. Wahn, Dr. Baker and Cynthia (my running partner of 20 years).

To my mother and sisters (twin Karen, Patty, and Jacque) who didn't ruin my self-esteem when I was overweight and who taught me unconditional love and positive role modeling!

To my colleagues at the University of San Diego Hahn School of Nursing and Health Science for the Professorship Award, which made it possible for me to complete this project!

To Dr. Jennings and my dear friend Jane who is smiling down from above for their love and encouragement which is why I selected a career in nursing!

To my patients who continuously teach me about challenges to become fit!

I dedicate this book in memory of my father, Richard Shadle, who encouraged me to engage in a lifetime of education!

INTRODUCTION

The book is divided into four parts:

PART ONE: THE WHOLE TRUTH ABOUT HABITS AND HEALTH

In the beginning, we will look at common health problems that face us today and how lifestyle choices are repeatedly the culprits. In Chapter 1 you become aware of habits that lead to problems and learn guidelines for good health. You can compare your daily food choices and exercise level with recommended guidelines to learn if what you're doing is keeping you strong and healthy and which habits could lead to future health problems. Or, you'll find out you're the optimum of good health and give this book to a friend!! In Chapter 2 you can test your eating and exercise habits. You can also measure your body mass index (BMI), waist measurement and evaluate your risks for disease. These simple quizzes will make you aware if you're already on track (hurray) or if you have room for improvement.

PART TWO: WHAT DO WE EAT?

In Chapter 3 you'll learn what and how much you need to eat. Specialty diets usually tell you what to eat and how much, but when you're designing your own food plan it's confusing to put it all together. This chapter discusses calorie needs and caloric density to make you aware of your body's actual energy needs. The Food Guide Pyramid chart as well as the Mayo Clinic Pyramid chart (a modification of the traditional Food Guide Pyramid) are included. You will learn how to determine your daily servings of different foods, whether your goal is to maintain or lose weight.

Chapter 4 covers the major nutrients: protein, carbohydrates, and fats, and how much you need of each. At the end of the chapter, you can evaluate your current food choices in relation to healthy guidelines.

Chapter 5 focuses on how to follow a vegetarian diet without missing out on major nutrients. Chapter 6 provides you with information on how to get the most energy from the foods you eat. This information will be particularly helpful if you have low energy, are overweight, or at risk for diabetes. A glycemic index is included for common foods.

Chapter 7 provides specific guidelines for readers with high cholesterol and triglycerides. Chapter 8 focuses on fiber. This information is included because of my experience with patients who are plagued with constipation, thinking they are eating a high-fiber diet only to find it's actually low in fiber.

PART THREE: EATING ON THE GO

Chapter 9 gives you guidelines for planning healthy quick meals in advance and actual food plans! Tips on what to keep on hand in your cupboards and sample eating plans are provided. You'll be ready to take this shopping list to the grocery store. My favorite recipes are shared in Chapter 10.

PART FOUR: OVERWEIGHT? HOW TO LOSE IT!

Chapter 11 reviews my 10-step approach to successful weight loss and provides you with the same information that I use one-on-one with patients in private practice. Specific, simple guidelines to set weight-loss and behavioral goals, design a personalized eating guide, and evaluate your progress are listed.

PART ONE

THE WHOLE TRUTH ABOUT HABITS AND HEALTH

Chapter One

Bull's-eye: Target Health

Does it really matter what we eat? After all, we've had low-fat, low-calorie food choices for years, and yet people are still overweight and dying of heart disease. Or is the problem that we have options, but we don't make the best choices? Why do so many things get in the way of living and eating for a healthy lifestyle?

Think about the common health problems that your friends or relatives talk about when you are together. (Or maybe you avoid this discussion?) Then think about the relationship between lifestyle, everyday habits, and health.

The major health problems—heart disease, diabetes, hypertension, and obesity—are affected by what we put in our mouth and by how much we move our bodies.

- According to American Heart Association statistics, heart disease killed 945,836 Americans in 2000. Compare that number to other major causes of death: cancer, 553,091; accidents, 97,900; Alzheimer's disease, 49,558; and HIV (AIDS), 14,478. Can you do something to prevent heart disease? Yes, through your diet and lifestyle. Cancer? Yes, through your diet. Accidents? Yes, through your lifestyle. Alzheimer's? The answers are not yet clear. HIV? Yes, through lifestyle changes as well.
- According to American Diabetes Association statistics, there are approximately **20 million Americans who are diabetic.** The unfortunate thing is almost half of these people don't know it! The life expectancy of diabetics can be shortened by one third. However, early diagnosis and lifestyle changes can substantially increase life expectancy. This disease is the ***third leading killer in this country—behind heart***

disease and cancer. The prevalence of diabetes is particularly high in minority populations including American Indians, Hispanic/Latino Americans and African Americans. Can you do something to prevent diabetes? In most cases, **yes**—especially with Type 2 diabetes.

- High blood pressure is another silent but deadly health problem that many people don't know about. *It is estimated that one in four U.S. adults have high blood pressure.* Uncontrolled high blood pressure can lead to stroke, heart attack, heart failure, or kidney failure. Can you do something to prevent high blood pressure? **Yes!**
- *Obesity now affects between 55% and 61% of our population.* More than 300,000 Americans die prematurely each year from obesity-related disease. Obesity costs the United States $120 BILLION each year.

Can you do something to prevent obesity? **Yes.**

There are actually pretty simple lifestyle and eating modifications to prevent the above problems. Is it a surprise to learn that nearly 40% of adults never exercise? Our health conditions are a result of our lifestyles. The good thing is that we can all choose to do something about the behaviors that affect our health! Part of the answer, as you have heard many times, is eating a healthy diet and exercising.

Education can play an important role in making changes. First we need to be made aware of factors that will influence our health. Then we need to make the personal choices! This book was written to provide you with the information and motivation to make healthy choices in your food choices as well as your lifestyle choices.

Look at the Dietary Guidelines for Americans listed below. Are you already achieving these goals? To reduce risk of diseases that are diet-related, you need to:

Aim for Fitness

Target your healthy weight. (Chapter 2 will provide that number if you're not sure.)

Be physically active every day. (Recent guidelines recommend a minimum of 60 minutes per day.)

Build a Health Base

Let the food pyramid guide your food choices. (We'll cover this in Chapter 3.) Fats and sugars can be consumed in tiny amounts. Eat a variety of grains daily, especially whole grains (cereal, whole grain breads, muffins, or rice). Eat a variety of fruits and vegetables daily. (Aim for at least five to seven servings a day.)

For safety, keep foods in the refrigerator and food cabinets.

Choose Sensibly

Choose a diet that is low in saturated fat (the white grease that is left after you've cooked a hamburger) and cholesterol and moderate in total fat. Meats are sources of saturated fat, as are many packaged snacks. Fruits and vegetables do not have fat in them.

Choose beverages and foods that are low in sugar: A 12-ounce soda has 12 teaspoons of sugar!

Choose and prepare foods with less salt. You get plenty of sodium in your diet without adding extra salt.

If you drink alcoholic beverages, do so in moderation.

These are pretty basic, helpful tips. If my patients followed even half of these guidelines, I probably wouldn't see them in the clinic to manage their diabetes, high cholesterol, or high blood pressure.

EXAMPLES OF LIFESTYLE HABITS THAT CAN HELP RESOLVE HEALTH PROBLEMS

Health Problem	Helpful Lifestyle Habits
1. Obesity	Plan an activity five times a week for at least 20 minutes.

Eat foods low in fat.
Limit junk food (candy, sodas, cookies) to control calories.
Eat fruits, vegetables and whole grains.

2. **Heart disease** Control blood pressure with diet and daily exercise
Don't smoke.
Eat high-fiber, low-fat foods.
Watch salt intake.

3. **Diabetes** Keep weight in normal range.
Eat a healthy diet (low fat, low sugar, high fiber).
Exercise 30 minutes at least five days a week.

Why is it so difficult to lead a healthy lifestyle? Let's get the excuses out of the way now.

1. Fast food is readily available and easy. (Response: Fine. There are healthy choices at most fast food restaurants—choose appropriately!)

2. TV makes junk food look delicious and fun to eat. (Response: That is correct. That's why it accompanies morning cartoons. You'll notice there is little reference to healthy foods!)

3. Our friends eat burgers and fries, cheese and nachos. (Response: I don't suggest you never eat a burger again—eating in moderation is the key.)

4. Our culture focuses on food to celebrate. (Response: Celebrations can include healthy foods!)

5. Our family always grabs something quick and fast. (Response: It's just as easy to grab "planned" healthy snacks and meals.)

6. We have too many activities and not enough time to exercise. (Response: Incorporate exercise into your daily

activities. ***Remember, not exercising is a big risk factor for heart disease.***)

7. We are too busy to sit down to eat. (Response: Families miss out by not taking this time together. Do you really know what's going on in your child's and spouse's life?)

8. We don't have money to buy "fancy" foods. (Response: Fresh fruits and vegetables aren't "fancy"—just healthy!)

9. Our children won't eat fruits and vegetables. (Response: Slowly incorporate them in small servings throughout their diet.)

10. We're lazy. (Response: Let's change that self-talk too!)

Sometimes families have to re-examine what's important in their lives. When I talk with a family unable to find one night a week to have fun together or to plan a meal together, I wonder about the family's stress level. Even small lifestyle changes can make a big difference between being normal weight and overweight, and between good health and poor health. For example, a 15- to 20-minute walk every day will burn about 150 calories. If you add that to your daily routine, that would total a 15-pound weight loss in one year! While your child is at baseball practice, walk around the field. Put the baby in the stroller and walk a couple of times a day. Take your children for a walk with you after dinner.

Look at these examples of changes that have occurred during the past 20 years. We are eating out more and, as a result of our food choices and lifestyle choices, our health has suffered.

1980s	**2000s**
$6 billion spent on fast food	$100 billion spent on fast food
1,000 fast food restaurants	23,000 fast food restaurants
75% of meals eaten at home	Majority of meals eaten outside of the home

one-third of mothers with young children work	two-thirds of mothers with young children work
Children eat 5 servings of fruit and vegetables	20% of children eat 5 servings of fruit and vegetables

ACTIVITY HABITS

Here are examples of how activity levels are changing in our country.
* Almost two-thirds of 9- to 13-year-olds participate in NO organized physical activity outside of school
* In fifth grade, *only* 50% of schools require physical education (PE) classes
* In tenth grade, only 9.5% of schools require any PE classes
* Even in SUNNY California, only 24% of the state's fifth, seventh, and ninth graders met minimal physical-education standards in 2002

Is it any surprise the rate of childhood obesity has doubled in the past 20 years?

FAMILY TIME

The Carole family came to me for help with their habits. The parents, in their 30s, have two children, 8 and 13 years old. The family was concerned because they were all gaining weight. Up to this point, the family members had been pretty healthy, although extended family members were on medications for high cholesterol and blood pressure. Everyone agreed they'd like to be healthy.

We looked at the possible culprits together. Common foods being consumed in their household included sugary cereals, 2% milk, desserts after dinner, school meals consisting of cheese and pepperoni pizza, and only a rare consumption of vegetables. Neither child was active after school, and the parents felt they weren't able to fit exercise into their busy schedules. On the positive side, they watched very little TV (one show a night) and, most important, they were all willing to make changes. Their family plan included;

1. taking a healthy lunch to school three to four times a week.
2. selecting cereals with less sugar.
3. keeping a fruit bowl in the kitchen for snacks, filled especially with fruit the children like.
4. working on being more active and planning at least one family activity together on weekends, like hiking or biking.

Even if you have a family history of obesity, heart disease, cancer, or diabetes, you don't need to give up or say, "I can't do anything about it." In the next chapter, you'll have the opportunity to evaluate your habits and weight.

Chapter Highlight: A weight loss of only 10% of your body weight is often enough to result in decreasing your cholesterol level, blood sugar, and blood pressure. If you weigh 180 pounds and lose 18 pounds during the next year, you'll lose inches, have more energy, and lower your risk of diabetes. In one national study on diabetes, a 7% loss of body weight resulted in a 58% decrease in risk of diabetes. Now, that's a big deal!

Chapter Two

Habitually Healthy

In this section, you will have the opportunity to answer questions to help you evaluate your habits. You can't set goals until you know your strengths and weaknesses! Eating and exercise habits affect your weight and health. If you or your family receives a high score, chances are you're already striving to take good care of yourself. For example, parents who buy healthy foods for the house and eat meals together have a good chance of having normal-weight children. And most active parents have active children. In contrast, parents who bring home and consume sugary cereals, Doritos, doughnuts, and regular sodas have children who habitually eat junk food and prefer junk food. Parents who keep healthy snacks in the house, like low-fat cheese, whole-wheat crackers, fresh fruit, and ready-to-eat veggies are most likely to have children who eat these foods. Parents who watch four hours of TV a day usually have children who report that they watch three to four hours a day. Get the picture? You are important to the health of your family.

Circle the points that correlate with your family's usual eating habits.

Food Check   **Points**

1. a. We drink two to three servings of nonfat milk or yogurt daily.   5
   b. We use regular cheeses and whole milk.   0
2. a. We eat high-fiber breads and cereals.   5
   b. We eat white bread and sugary cereals.   0
3. a. We eat chicken, fish, and lean meats three to four times a week.   5
   b. We eat hamburgers and fast food three to four times a week.   0

4. a. We eat at least three servings of fruits a day.	5
b. We drink juices and sodas almost daily.	0
5. a. We eat at least two cups of vegetables a day.	5
b. We rarely eat vegetables.	0
c. We eat vegetables with butter.	0
6. a. We rarely eat junk food.	5
b. We eat junk food daily.	0
7. a. We eat when we are hungry.	5
b. We eat when we are bored, upset, or to celebrate.	0
8. a. We stop eating when we are satisfied.	5
b. We stop eating when we are full.	0
9. a. We have a balance of rest and activity in our life.	5
b. We are always tired or stressed out.	0
10. a. We have supportive people in our life.	5
b. We feel alone a lot and don't have anyone to talk to.	0

Total points _____

40-50: You're looking really good!
30-39: You're not far behind the strong ones!
20-29: It's time for a plan!
Less than 20: Look out, doctor. Here we come!

    Circle one or two areas that you'd like to change to improve your score. Place a star next to each habit that you feel you are already excelling in.

Exercise Check	**Points**
1. We exercise at least once a week.	0
2. We exercise at least three to five times a week for 30 to 45 minutes.	5
3. We do some exercises (e.g., sit-ups, push-ups, weightlifting) to keep our bodies strong at least three times a week.	5
4. All of the members in our family are physically active.	5
5. No one exercises regularly right now.	0

6. We think exercise is important to be healthy.   5
7. We don't have time to exercise in our family.   0

Total points _____

15–20: Way to go! You're really on target!!
10: You're halfway there! Set some goals!
Less than 10: Time for a reality check. Is health important to you?

Add your scores, and rate your family's exercise habits. Circle one or two areas that you'd like to change to improve your score. Place a star next to habits that you're already happy with!

To evaluate your risk for health problems based on what you weigh, it's important to check three key measurements:
1. body mass index (BMI)
2. waist circumference
3. risk factors for diseases or conditions associated with obesity

BMI is a measure of your weight in relation to your height. BMI is used to evaluate overweight and obesity. Some very muscular people may meet the criteria for obesity, although they are not obese. Waist circumference and waist-hip ratio may also be used to evaluate obesity. Waist circumference measures how much fat is around your middle. Together, this information helps you know your risk for developing diseases associated with obesity. The goal is to avoid developing health problems by taking early action.

BMI calculates if you're underweight, normal, overweight, or obese. Find your height in the left column and then your body weight to the right. Then go to the top of the page and find the number associated with your height and weight. That is your BMI. Check to see if your BMI is normal or overweight.

Body Mass Index for Adults

To use the table, find the appropriate height in the left-hand column labeled Height. Move across to a given weight. The number at the top of the column is the BMI at that height and weight. have been rounded off.

BMI	19	20	21	22	23	24	25	26	27	28	29	30	31	32	33	34	35
Height (inches)	Body Weight (pounds)																
58	91	96	100	105	110	115	119	124	129	134	138	143	148	153	158	162	167
59	94	99	104	109	114	119	124	128	133	138	143	148	153	158	163	168	173
60	97	102	107	112	118	123	128	133	138	143	148	153	158	163	168	174	179
61	100	106	111	116	122	127	132	137	143	148	153	158	164	169	174	180	185
62	104	109	115	120	126	131	136	142	147	153	158	164	169	175	180	186	191
63	107	113	118	124	130	135	141	146	152	158	163	169	175	180	186	191	197
64	110	116	122	128	134	140	145	151	157	163	169	174	180	186	192	197	204
65	114	120	126	132	138	144	150	156	162	168	174	180	186	192	198	204	210
66	118	124	130	136	142	148	155	161	167	173	179	186	192	198	204	210	216
67	121	127	134	140	146	153	159	166	172	178	185	191	198	204	211	217	223
68	125	131	138	144	151	158	164	171	177	184	190	197	203	210	216	223	230
69	128	135	142	149	155	162	169	176	182	189	196	203	209	216	223	230	236
70	132	139	146	153	160	167	174	181	188	195	202	209	216	222	229	236	243
71	136	143	150	157	165	172	179	186	193	200	208	215	222	229	236	243	250
72	140	147	154	162	169	177	184	191	199	206	213	221	228	235	242	250	258
73	144	151	159	166	174	182	189	197	204	212	219	227	235	242	250	257	265
74	148	155	163	171	179	186	194	202	210	218	225	233	241	249	256	264	272
75	152	160	168	176	184	192	200	208	216	224	232	240	248	256	264	272	279
76	156	164	172	180	189	197	205	213	221	230	238	246	254	263	271	279	287

Adapted from "Clinical Guidelines on the Identification, Evaluation, and Treatment of Overweight and Obesity in Adults: The Evidence Report"

Classification of Overweight and Obesity

	BMI (kg/m2)
Underweight	<18.5
Normal	18.5-24.9
Overweight	25-29.9
Obesity	30-34.9
Extreme obesity	40+

You can also do your own calculation if you don't find your height or weight on the scale. This formula is appropriate for children as well. BMI can be calculated using pounds and inches with this equation:

$$BMI = \frac{\text{Weight in Pounds}}{(\text{Height in inches}) \times (\text{Height in inches})} \times 703$$

For example, a person who weighs 220 pounds and is six feet three inches tall has a BMI of 27.5.

$$\frac{220 \text{ lbs.}}{(75 \text{ inches}) \times (75 \text{ inches})} \times 703 = 27.5$$

Note, there are some limitations in evaluating your BMI if you are an athlete or an older person. It can overestimate body fat in athletes and those with a muscular build. It may underestimate body fat in persons who have lost muscle mass, such as older persons.

BMI is also used to evaluate if children are "at risk" for being overweight. Your pediatrician will make this determination at your annual checkups, or you may calculate your child's BMI. (See BMI charts for boys and girls in the Appendix.) The Web site at the Centers for Disease Control also provides charts to determine children's BMI. If the BMI is above the 85th percentile, they're considered "at risk" of being overweight. Above the 95th percentile is considered overweight. More detailed strategies are discussed in the section on weight management in Chapter 11.

Next, check your waist measurement. Wrap a tape measure snugly around your waist. If you are a male with a waist of 40 inches or greater, or a female with a waist of 35 inches or greater, you are at increased risk for diabetes, hypertension, and cardiovascular diseases. Check your hip measurement, and divide the waist measurement by the hip measurement. For females, a ratio of 0.81 or less is a healthy zone. For males, a ratio of 1.01 or less is a healthy waist-hip ratio. For example, a male with a waist of 42 and hips of 42½ inches has a ratio of 0.99. The 42-inch waist measurement is a risk factor.

There are other risk factors to consider, or you may already have existing conditions that could put you at increased risk for health problems. For example, having a high cholesterol level is a risk for heart disease, heart attack or stroke. A lipid profile is a blood test that will tell you about your total cholesterol (TC), high density lipid cholesterol (HDL-C), low density lipid cholesterol (LDL-C) and triglycerides. Just remember that LDL-C is the bad cholesterol that carries cholesterol to artery walls, HDL is the good cholesterol because it helps remove cholesterols from artery walls. High triglyceride levels are another risk factor for coronary heart disease (CHD). Factors that can elevate triglycerides include cigarette smoking, being overweight, physical inactivity, high carbohydrate diets and some diseases. I talk more about these in Chapter 7. Be aware, but not frightened. Risk factors can be reduced when people make positive changes in their habits.

Risk Factors Besides Being Overweight

High blood pressure (hypertension)	optimal is less than 120/80
High LDL cholesterol (bad cholesterol)	optimal is below 100
Low HDL cholesterol (good cholesterol)	optimal is 60 and above
High blood glucose (sugar)	optimal is less than 90
High triglycerides	normal is below 150

Family history of early heart disease (before age 50)
Physical inactivity (exercise three or fewer days a week)
Cigarette smoking

Adapted from National Lipid Cholesterol Education Council, Winter 2002/2003

Summarize your results below:

My BMI is _____. "Circle one" - I am underweight, normal, overweight, or obese.

My waist circumference is _____. I'm in a range that is not considered at risk _____. I am in a range that is considered at risk _____.

Risk factors for family members: _____

Family members who have a normal BMI and waist measurement, and no risk factors:_____
_____.

Family members who have abnormal blood-test values: _____.

If you don't know your blood-test values as listed in the table, make an appointment with your health care professional and find out. This information will help you recognize whether or not you have risk factors for heart disease and diabetes. If you do, you can make the changes necessary to improve your health.

FAMILY TIME

The Smiths came to me to help them with their eating and exercise habits. Here's their evaluation and plan:

Eating score: 20 (room for improvement)

Plan: Consume less heavy foods, like pizza and desserts, at dinner.

Exercise score: 10 (no one exercised consistently)

Plan: Keep a calendar of everyone's weekly minutes of exercise.

Begin with a goal of 150 minutes per week. Work up to 60 minutes a day, if possible. A pedometer will help you track your distance. Aim for 10,000 steps per day.

Example of family evaluation:

Mother's BMI: 27 (overweight); waist: 35 (at risk)

Father's BMI: 32 (obese); waist: 42 (at risk)

15-year-old girl's BMI: 26 (overweight); waist/hip ratio: 0.81 (okay)

9-year-old son's BMI: 26 (overweight); waist/hip ratio: 0.90 (okay)

Risk factors: father has high cholesterol; family is physically inactive

Plan: Everyone will work on increasing activity level and record daily steps from their pedometers on a calendar. Since everyone is overweight, the family agreed to cut out desserts and replace them with lower-fat items, such as nonfat yogurt and sliced fruit, and to eat fast food no more than once a week.

Now that you've completed your self-assessment, how do you feel? Elated, or ready for a little more action? It can be fun—you decide on the changes you want to make and the pace. You can take it slow or a little faster. Whatever pleases you. Decide on one change. Be specific about what you want to accomplish. Record it on your calendar. Example: *I want to be more active. I will walk 30 minutes four to five times a week and record my minutes on my calendar.*

Chapter Highlight: Take the challenge. If you're not currently eating healthy foods or exercising, obtain a baseline of your labs from your doctor (blood pressure, resting pulse, blood sugar, lipid panel, and a fitness test, if possible). The fitness test can be as simple as seeing how many sit-ups you can do. Or, time how long it takes you to walk or run one mile, whichever you can do. Try sitting on the floor and see how far you can stretch to reach your toes. Give yourself six weeks of reduced fat eating and regular exercise. Then repeat your blood work and fitness test, and see the improvements!

PART TWO

WHAT DO WE EAT?

Chapter Three

Food Choices: What and How Much?

A frequent question families ask is, What should we eat and how much? My first response is to share a simple food summary guide that lists foods as "free," "light," "heavy," or "junk." Ideally, most of your choices should come from the free and light food categories, with fewer choices from the heavy and junk food categories. The food summary lists **FREE FOODS** as very low in calories and sugar. Examples are green beans, lettuce, and tomatoes. Fat is minimal in the free group.

The **LIGHT FOODS** are also low in calories, fat, and sugar. They include beans, nonfat milk, light-meat chicken, and fruit. Thirty percent or fewer calories come from fat.

HEAVY FOODS are higher in fat and sugar, so you shouldn't eat them as often. Examples include peanut butter, sweetened cereals, hot dogs, and macaroni and cheese. The fat intake in this group is between 30 and 50% of the total calories, and you will find a higher amount of sugar in these types of foods.

JUNK FOODS include foods that are almost all fat or sugar, such as mayonnaise, butter, Kool-Aid, honey, cookies, ice cream, fruit drinks, granola bars, and Jell-O. More than 50% of the calories in these foods come from fat and/or sugar; some junk foods are 100% fat or sugar.

Families who are overweight include too many heavy and junk foods in their diet. The bodies of children often can't grow properly if they eat too many of these types of food because junk foods lack vitamins and minerals. You may include some junk foods but not often.

I hope the following Food Summary is a helpful guide.

FOOD SUMMARY

FREE FOODS			
artichokes	dill pickles	mineral water	sour pickles
asparagus	eggplant	mushrooms	soy sauce
bamboo shoots	flavorings	mustard	spices
broccoli	garlic	onion powder	sprouts
broth	green beens	onions	summer squash
brussel sprouts	green onions	peppers	tabasco sauce
cabbage	greens	popcorn, plain	tea
carrots	herbs	radishes	tomatoes
cauliflower	horseradish	salad dressing	tomato juice
celery	jicama	(no oil)	vegetable juice
cinnamon	lemon	sauerkraut	water
coffee	lettuce	Soda, diet	water chestnuts
cucumbers	limes	soda water	zuchinni

LIGHT FOODS			
apples	cereal,	grapes	raisins
applesauce,	unsweetened	grits	rice
canned w/o	cheese,	hamburger bun	rice cakes
sugar	reduced fat	lentils	spaghetti
apricots	cherries	meat, lean red	split peas
bananas	chicken, light	all fat removed	strawberries
bagel (plain)	meat, no skin	milk, non-fat	sweet potatoes
blackberries	clear soup	milk, low-fat	tangerines
black-eyed peas	cottage cheese	nectarines	tortillas
beens, dried	low fat	oranges	tuna,
beans, refried	crackers, low-	papaya	canned in water
biscuits	fat	peaches	turkey, light
bran	english muffins	pears	meat no skin
bread	edamane beans	peas	vegetable soups
bread sticks	fish	pineapple	watermelon
buttermilk	fruit, canned in	plums	winter squash
cantalope	water or juice	potatoes	yogurt,
	grapefruit	prunes	plain low-fat

Food Choices: What and How Much?

HEAVY FOODS			
almonds	corn bread	hash browns	potato salad
applesauce, sweetened	cottage cheese creamed	macaroni & cheese	pudding stuffing
avocado	crackers, high fat	macaroni salad	sunflower seeds
cereal, sweetened (5 gms sugar or >)	cream soups	meat, red	taco shells, fried
	eggs	milk, chocolate	tofu
cheese	fish, fried	milk, ice	tuna, in oil
chicken, fried	fish sticks breaded	milk, lowfat 2%	turkey hot dogs
chicken or turkey dark meat	french toast	milk, whole	vegetables in in sauce
chicken or turkey with skin	fries	muffins	waffles
	fruit, canned in syrup	pancakes	yogurt, flavored low-fat
chili		peanut butter	
coconut	fruit rolls	peanuts	yogurt, frozen low-fat
	granola	pizza	
		popcorn, buttered	

JUNK FOODS			
bacon	croissants	jelly	salt
beer	doughnuts	kool-aid	sausage
butter	fruit drinks	liquor	shakes
candy	granola bars	margarine	sherbert
candy cereal	candy bars	mayonnaise	sodas, regular
cakes	gravy	oil	sour cream
chips	gum	olives	sugar
chocolate	half and half	pastries	sweet pickles
chocolate topping	honey	pies	syrup
cookies	hot dogs	popsicles	tartar sauce
cream cheese	ice cream	salad dressing	whipped cream
cream sauce	jam	salami	wine
	jello		

Reprinted with permission from Bob Mellin, *SHAPEDOWN*, Balboa Publishing.

Circle the foods you've eaten in the past week. Check which categories have the most circles. If you find a lot of circles in the heavy and junk food areas, start to change these habits by not buying those foods as often. Remember, a heavy and junk food diet is <u>not</u> healthy for anyone. Eventually, too many of these types of food will raise your cholesterol, increase your potential for being overweight, and can cause cavities!

Besides being aware of the types of food you eat, it is helpful to consider how many calories are in different foods. This is sometimes referred to as "caloric density." Note the difference in high- versus low-calorie dense foods from one cup of various foods.

Food Choices: What and How Much?

Caloric Density of Foods (serving size = one cup)

FOOD	KCAL	FOOD	KCAL
Canola oil	1925	Macaroni, cooked	190
Butter	1630	White rice, cooked	180
Margarine	1630	Clam chowder	180
Roasted trail mix	1040	Chardonnay wine	176
Chocolate candy	860	Tomato soup, milk	175
Peanuts	840	Grape juice	165
Whipping cream	820	Whole milk	150
Sunflower seeds	810	Apricot nectar	145
Jelly beans	807	Sweet corn	130
Cashew nuts	785	Oatmeal, breakfast	130
White sugar	770	Orange juice	120
Granola	520	Low-fat milk	120
Parmesan cheese	455	Apple juice	120
Seedless raisins	420	Peas	110
Ice cream (16% fat)	350	Total cereal	110
Cheese, ricotta, skim milk	340	Orange	90
Spaghetti, tomato/meat	330	Nonfat milk	85
Cream, half-and-half	315	Raspberries	70
Ice cream (11% fat)	270	Peaches, raw	55
Turkey, no skin	265	Strawberries	55
Cottage cheese (4% fat)	235	Spinach, cooked	45

Low-fat yogurt w/ fruit	230	Broccoli, cooked	40
Red kidney beans	230	Green beans	35
Ground beef (10% fat)	224	Cauliflower, raw	31
Whole lentils, cooked	210	Celery	20
		Lettuce, raw	5

Foods in the left column have a higher caloric density than the foods in the right column.
When trying to lose weight, emphasize your selection of foods with the lower caloric density.

Here's a quick verbal check used to review nutritional habits. Write your response next to each question.
Do you
- eat three to four pieces of fruit daily?
- have at least three servings of milk, yogurt or cheese daily?
- have two cups of veggies daily?
- eat two servings of lean meat, chicken, fish, or legumes daily?
- include four or more servings of whole-grain breads and cereals daily?
- limit your fat intake?
- avoid junk food?

If you answered "yes" to all of the questions, bravo! If you responded with "no" answers to the questions, take a look at what you are missing or eating too much of—for example, eating no vegetables or not limiting your fat intake. It's important to be aware of where you're getting too much or too little, and then take the steps necessary to improve your health.

How much to eat?

Unfortunately, food is not always looked at as fuel or energy. How active are you? Do you sit most of the day, or are you up and running or on your feet eight to ten hours a day? Are you young or old? All of these factors affect how much food (fuel/energy) you need. Can you pinch an inch around your waist? If you can pinch more than an inch, chances are you are eating too much and would benefit from smaller amounts. Use the Food Guide Pyramid chart to check the servings you have each day. Let's review what a serving is. For example, many store-bought bagels are really equal to having three to four slices of bread, even though you might think it's one serving! An average serving of bread is about 80 calories, fruit is 60 calories, nonfat milk products are about 90 to 110 calories, and meat ranges from 35 to 100 calories per ounce, depending on if it's very lean or high in fat.

How to Use the Food Guide Pyramid

How many servings do you need each day?

What counts as a serving?	Children ages 2 to 6 Women, some older adults (1,600 calories)	Older children teen girls, active women, most men (2,200 calories)	Teen boys active men (2,800 calories)
Grains Group (Bread, Cereal, Rice, and Pasta)— Especially whole grain • 1 slice of bread • about 1 cup of ready-to-eat cereal • ½ cup cooked cereal, rice or pasta	6	9	11
Vegetable Group • 1 cup of raw leafy vegetables • ½ cup of other vegetables, cooked or raw • ¾ cup vegetable juice	3	4	5
Fruit Group • 1 med apple, banana, orange, or pear • ½ cup chopped, cooked, or canned fruit • ¾ cup fruit juice	2	3	4
Milk, Yogurt, and Cheese Group Preferably fat-free or low-fat • 1 cup milk** or yogurt • 1½ oz of natural cheese (like cheddar) • 2 oz processed cheese (like American)	2 or 3*	2 or 3*	2 or 3*

Food Choices: What and How Much?

Meat and Beans Group (Meat, Poultry, Fish, Dry Beans, Eggs, and Nuts)	2, for a total of 5 ounces	2, for a total of 5 ounces	3, for a total of 7 ounces

Preferably lean or low fat
- 2-3 oz of cooked lean meat, poultry, or fish
  These count as 1 oz of meat:
- ½ cup cooked dry beans or tofu
- 2½ oz soy burger
- 1 egg
- 2 tbsp peanut butter
- 1/3 cup of nuts

Adapted from United States Department of Agriculture
*older children and teens ages 9 to 18 years and adults over age 50 need 3 servings daily; others need two
** This includes lactose free and lactose reduced milk products. Soy based beverages with added calcium are an option for those who prefer a non-dairy source of calcium.

FAMILY TIME

Here's a sample plan for a 40-year-old woman who works out four days a week. We'll compare her food intake to the pyramid guide.

Breakfast

1 banana = 1 fruit serving
1 cup nonfat milk = 1 milk serving
1 slice whole-wheat bread = 1 bread serving
½ cup whole-grain cereal = 1 bread serving
1 tsp margarine

> **Lunch**
>
> 3 oz chicken salad = greater than 1 meat serving
> 3 small breadsticks = 2 bread servings
> 2 cups mixed lettuce greens = 2 vegetable servings
> 2 tbsp light salad dressing
> iced tea
>
> **Snack**
>
> 1 cup carrot sticks = 2 vegetable serving
> 1 med apple = 1 fruit serving
> 1 nonfat yogurt = 1 milk serving
>
> **Dinner**
>
> 3 oz grilled salmon = greater than 1 meat serving
> 1 cup brown or wild rice = 2 bread servings
> ½ cup carrots, cooked = 1 vegetable serving
> 2 cups green salad with chopped pear = 2 vegetable servings and 1 fruit serving
> 1 tbsp olive oil, flaxseed, or high-oleic safflower oil
>
> <u>Total servings = 6 breads, 7 vegetables, 3 fruit, 2 milk, 6 oz protein</u>

EVALUATION: 1. As a female, she still needs another serving of calcium, or she could supplement with 300 milligrams of calcium. 2. If she exercises five or six days a week, another recommendation would be two to three more bread servings. 3. Otherwise, the intake of fruits, vegetables, and whole grains looks balanced.

When comparing food records with the pyramid, look for obvious gaps such as drinking no milk, eating twice the amount of protein needed, eating too few servings of fruits or vegetables, and eating hidden or excessive added fat.

One of the newer food pyramids for weight-conscious people was developed at the Mayo Clinic based on experiences with patients who wanted to lose weight (see Web Resources).

The five-level pyramid is designed to help you lose or maintain a healthy weight, and it focuses on unlimited amount of fruits and whole vegetables.

Level One: Fruits and vegetables. A minimum of four servings of fruits and vegetables are recommended daily. For example: ½ cup of juice or one small serving of fruit

Level Two: Whole grains. Four to eight servings a day are recommended. For example: ½ cup of cereal

Level Three: Protein/dairy. Three to seven servings are recommended daily. For example: ⅓ cup of beans, 3 oz of meat or fish or 1 cup of milk

Level Four: Fat. Three to five servings are recommended daily. For example: 1 tsp of oil or 1 tbsp of nuts

Level Five: Sweets. Keep this serving to a small sampling, and do not consume more than 525 calories per week from this level.

The pyramids are quite similar in recommendations. Drastically changing your diet is difficult and not necessary. Make one change per month; that will simplify the process for you!

The Food Guide Pyramid is helpful for checking serving sizes and recommendations for most ages. Start by keeping a record of your food intake, and compare your servings of grains, vegetables, fruit, milk, meat, and beans to the numbers shown for children, women, active women, men, and teen boys.

Here's an example of a simple way to assess types of food and food groups using the Food Summary.

- Begin by checking to see what types of food you are eating.
- Look at how many food servings of milk, meat, fruit/vegetables, and grains you're eating.
- Fats aren't included, but you'll be able to detect them under the heavy and junk food categories.

Food Item	serving	free	light	heavy	junk	milk	meat	fruit	veg	grain	other
Cheerios	1 cup	X								2	
Sugar	1 tbsp				X						sugar
Low-fat milk	1 cup	X				1					
Apple	1	X			X			1			
Nachos Cheese	2 cup			X						4	
Spaghetti	2 cups	X								4	
Tomato sauce	½ cup	X							1		
Hagan Daaz ice cream	1 cup				X	1					fat

FAMILY TIME

What gets in the way of following the pyramid guidelines? Here are some problems and possible solutions.

1. "My children are fussy." (Please remember that you are the parent. Unless you want to be a short-order cook, don't give in to pleading children.) If you don't bring a lot of junk food into the house, everyone will have an easier time making a decision about what they're going to eat. Pick one food-related habit to work on each month. For example, your children might be drinking unlimited amounts of juice. Try replacing the juices with fresh fruit and a glass of water. Most of us eat too little fiber to begin with, and juices are filled with sugar. Slice an apple, orange, or banana instead of pouring a large glass of juice. What takes longer to consume: apple juice, applesauce, or an apple? The apple will be more satisfying and filling because of the fiber and will also help prevent constipation!

2. Ethnic challenges. "We're Italian. We like our breads and pasta. It's common for us to have two to three servings of bread or rice at each meal." Enjoy your carbohydrates unless you are simply consuming too many and gaining weight. In that case, add some vegetables to your rice and pasta.

"We are Mexican-American—we like our tortillas!" No problem, as long as you aren't cooking your tortillas and beans in shortening and spreading butter all over them!

3. "We don't know what to follow." Atkins, the Zone Diet, or the South Beach Diet? It's so confusing. Don't diet—period. Don't do anything that you can't live with forever. Eat a variety of foods. Remember, you can gain weight eating too much of any of the food groups. Vegetarians can be overweight from too much fat from nuts and from too many servings of low-fat grains. (Remember, calories always count.) Atkins lovers' weight loss can come to a halt when they consume unlimited fats.

As far as the composition of your diet in relation to protein, carbohydrates, and fats, you can lose weight whether you're eating 45% or 65% carbohydrates. The bottom line is it still comes down to caloric intake and energy expenditure.

You now have an idea of the types and amount of food your body needs. I ask families with weight concerns, "Is it a problem with the TYPES of food you're eating or the AMOUNTS?" Think about it: it's easy to lighten up by eating less or by avoiding the heavy and junk foods. If food amounts are a problem, measure your food for a few days and do a reality check of how many servings you're really eating. Most people underestimate their intake and overestimate their activity level. Hmm!

Chapter Highlight: Fill your cupboard with free and light foods, and you'll see how easy it is to maintain a healthier lifestyle. If you get bored with what you're eating, spend an extra 20 minutes at the grocery store and try some new food choices. Keep it simple. Start with the Food Summary list to see how you're doing with your healthy choices.

And, remember, it's really not NATURAL or NECESSARY to give up an entire food group to reach your weight and health goals.

Chapter Four

Nutrient Basics: Protein, Carbohydrates, and Fats

I included this information because most people have not had a nutrition class since high school, college, or ever! The following recommendations are based on healthy, active individuals. Food gives us one or a combination of these aforementioned nutrients, and the following recommendations will help you understand your body's need versus the amounts consumed. For example, most young women will meet their protein needs with four ounces of lean chicken, fish, or meat and two cups of milk daily. In real life, they're often eating close to a half a pound or more of protein and drinking little or no milk.

> *Did you know: protein has four calories per gram, carbohydrates also have four calories per gram, fat has nine calories per gram, and alcohol has seven calories per gram.*

Because the body cannot store protein, it needs a new supply daily. Protein plays an important role in the growth and maintenance of body tissue and is composed of 22 different amino acids. Of the 22, eight must be provided by diet. The body can, with the necessary materials, make the other 14. In the United States, Dietary Reference Intakes have replaced the Recommended Dietary Allowance (RDA), although they are similar. Protein needs are based on age, weight, and general physical state.

The protein standard for adults is 0.8 g/kg of body weight or 0.4 grams per pound. This amounts to about 63 grams of protein per day for a man who weighs 174 pounds (79 kg) and 50 grams per day for a woman who weighs 138 pounds

(63 kg). (To change pounds to kilograms, divide your weight in pounds by 2.2).

It's possible to get the recommended amount of protein without eating meat. Other sources of protein include milk and cheese, beans and peas, tofu, rice, and nuts. Become familiar with common protein choices.

It's rare to find someone who is protein-deficient. Here's an example of how easy it is to meet your protein needs.

FAMILY TIME

This is the diet of a 10-year-old boy whose mother was concerned he was not getting enough protein:

Breakfast: 1 cup of Frosted Flakes, ½ cup of low-fat milk, 1 slice of white bread = 13 grams protein

Lunch: peanut butter sandwich with 2 slices of white bread, 1 cup of low-fat chocolate milk = 20 grams protein

Snack: 10 pretzel pieces, gummy bears = 5 grams protein

Dinner: 1 cup macaroni and cheese, ½ cup of green peas, soda = 17 grams protein

Total protein for the day is 55 grams.

The recommended intake for a 10-year-old is 34 grams of protein. This child had no problem eating enough protein. In fact, my recommendation would be for him to eat less protein and more fruits and vegetables.

Dietary Reference Intakes of Protein for Different Ages

Group	Protein grams/day
Infants 0-6 mo	9.1
7-12 mo	13.5
Children	
1 to 3 yrs	13
4 to 8 yrs	19
Males 9 to 13 yrs	34
14 to 18 yrs	52
19 to 70 yrs	56
31 to 70 yrs	56
Females	
9 to 13 yrs	34
14 to 70 yrs	46
Pregnancy	
<18 yrs	71
19-50 yrs	71
Lactation	71

Source: Food and Nutrition Information Center

Common Foods and Protein in Each

Milk Group	Amount	Protein Grams
Milk, whole	1 cup	9
Milk, skim	1 cup	9
Milk, soy	1 cup	7
Cheese	1 oz	6
Cottage cheese	½ cup	15
Yogurt	1 cup	8
Meat Group *Inc. Plants*		
Chicken breast	1 oz	8
Roast beef	1 oz	7
Tuna, canned	1 oz	7
Egg	1	6
Peanut butter	1 tbsp	4.5
Tofu	4 oz	11

Vegetable Group		
Lentils	½ cup	7
Baked beans	½ cup	7
Peas	½ cup	2
Carrots	½ cup	2
Potato	1 small	2
Fruit Group		
Banana	1	1
Apple	1	1
Grapefruit	½	1
Pear	1	1
Orange	1	1
Bread/Starch		
Bread, wheat	1 slice	3
Peas, split	½ cup	9
Macaroni	½ cup	9
Spaghetti	½ cup	3
Cereal	1 oz	2
Rice	1 cup cooked	4

Protein is readily available in foods. Looking at the big picture, *you ideally want about 12-15% of your calories from protein, 55-65% from carbohydrates and 20-30% from fat.* If you follow the pyramid guide recommendations discussed earlier, you'll be right on target.

Carbohydrates

These are the foods that make you "ready to go." They give you energy. Examples include: bread, cereal, rice and pasta, fruit, cookies, and candy. Most of your calories each day will come from this food group (hopefully minus the cookies and candy). Patients often claim they eat a lot of carbohydrates, and that would be normal since over 50% of your calories should come from carbohydrates.

You may have heard of simple and complex carbohydrates. Associate simple carbohydrates with sugar and complex carbohydrates with fiber. *Simple carbohydrates are easily digested and provide quick energy.* They are present in milk, fruits, and foods like soft drinks, jellies, candy, and ordinary table sugar. *Complex carbohydrates release energy more slowly and prevent large fluctuations in blood-sugar levels.* Complex carbohydrates are the better choice because a high concentration of sugar in large amounts, such as in a piece of cake, is more than the body can use at one time.

Good sources of complex carbohydrates include foods such as whole-wheat grains, beans and peas, and starches like potatoes. These foods are also higher in fiber, which makes you feel more satisfied. If you are constantly hungry after eating your sweet cereal or pancakes and syrup, you may find that eating complex carbohydrates for breakfast will be more satisfying and filling.

How do you know if you are eating too many carbohydrates? Take a look at how many servings from the bread group you're eating in a day. If you're overweight, you're eating too much of some food group. Here's an example of an overweight 16-year-old teen's food diary, with attention being given to the bread servings.

Breakfast: 2 cups Frosted Sugar Flakes, 1 cup low-fat milk, 1 piece of white bread toasted with butter and jelly = *5 bread servings*

Snack: 4 Oreo cookies = *2 bread servings*

Lunch: bean and cheese burrito = *2½ bread servings*

Snack: 2 oz potato chips and dip = *1 bread serving*

Dinner: French fries, cheeseburger with bun, low-fat milk = *4 bread servings*

Nutrient Basics: Protein, Carbohydrates, and Fats

She ate **14½ bread servings** in one day. That's higher than recommended on the food pyramid. Also note she didn't eat any fruit all day. She's filling up on simple carbohydrates.

You need to be an athlete to require 14½ bread servings. Since this teen is overweight, I'd recommend that she have four to eight servings from the bread group.

FAMILY TIME

Here's a sample of a revised food plan for the same 16-year-old. (The goal is to decrease her servings of breads/carbohydrates.)

Breakfast: 2 cups Sugar Frosted Flakes, 1 cup low-fat milk, 1 piece of white bread toasted with butter and jelly = 5 bread servings

Alternate: 1 cup whole wheat cheerios, 1 sliced apple, 1 cup nonfat milk = **1 bread serving**

Snack: 4 Oreo cookies = 2 bread servings

Alternate: 2 Oreo cookies and 1 tangerine= **1 bread serving**

Lunch: bean and cheese burrito = 2½ bread servings

Alternate: ½ turkey sandwich with baby carrots and light ranch dip, ½ banana, small nonfat yogurt = **1 bread serving**

Snack: 2 oz potato chips and dip = *1 bread serving*
Alternate: ½ cup applesauce

Dinner: French fries, cheeseburger with bun, low-fat milk = **4 bread servings**

Alternate: ½ baked potato, lean hamburger on whole-wheat bun, glass of nonfat milk, ½ banana = **3 bread servings**

*The revised diet has **6 bread servings** and 4 servings of fruit that are going to help her to feel satisfied.*

Choose whole-wheat buns, crackers, or brown rice. If you or your children are hungry all the time, it may be due to the kinds of foods you're eating. Some foods cause your blood sugar to rise quickly, then fall. Higher-fiber foods are less likely to do this.

Waist-watching women may also want to pay attention to their food choices if they're finding it difficult to lose weight. Here's an example of a gal on the run who was taking in more carbohydrates than she could burn. (The foods loaded with carbs will be noted.)

Breakfast: scone (loaded with fat, depending on where you buy them and the size; they can equal four to eight servings of bread)

Snack: caramel machiatto latte (the caramel is a source of carbohydrates that is often forgotten)

Lunch: 2 cups pasta salad with chicken (2 cups is like eating 4 bread servings), one pear

Snack: 4 cheese and peanut butter crackers (this is at least 2 bread servings)

Snack: 8 cups popcorn (3 cups is equal to one bread serving; watch the added butter)

Dinner: fish, 1 cup mashed potatoes (the potatoes equal about 2 servings of bread—not bad)

Unless you are hanging out at the gym for two hours a day, consider including more fresh fruit and vegetables in your meals. Enough about carbohydrates. They're not bad; they give you good energy. You just don't need huge amounts unless you're a mountain climber or very athletic.

For mothers: sometimes it's easier if you leave your little ones at home when you go to the store, or make it a point to shop the outer aisles. Better yet, just be a parent and call the shots on what you have in the house and in your cupboards! Don't forget to shop with a list!

Now about Cereals

This is a problem area for a lot of kids, and adults too. If you've eaten sugary cereals all your life, it's difficult to make the switch. Check the cereal labels and search for the added sugar. Look for no more than *five grams of sugar* (four grams is one teaspoon), no more than 200 milligrams of sodium, and at least two to three grams of fiber per serving (more fiber is okay) and 100% of the daily recommended values of folic acid. Other names for sugar that you may see on the label include sucrose, fructose, corn syrup, and maltodextrin.

Breakfast Foods Low in Sugar

Hot cereals (oatmeal, Cream of Wheat, Malt-O-Meal)
Kellogg's All-Bran
Kellogg's Corn Flakes
Kellogg's Product 19
Kellogg's Rice Krispies
Cheerios (regular and multigrain)
Corn Chex, Wheat Chex, Rice Chex
General Mills Wheaties
General Mills Fiber One
General Mills Total
Shredded Wheat
Puffed Kashi

Breakfast Foods High in Sugar

Cinnamon Toast Crunch
Cracklin' Oat Bran
Oatmeal Crisp with Raisins
Raisin Bran
Kellogg's Low Fat Granola with Raisins
Frosted Pop-Tarts
Cinnamon buns
Doughnuts

Here's a sampling of cereals and their sugar content.

Kellogg's Frosted Flakes	17 g	(over 4 tsp of sugar)
Raisin Bran	18 g	(almost 5 tsp of sugar)
Cap'n Crunch	15 g	(3 tsp of sugar)
Froot Loops	12 g	(3 tsp of sugar)
Product 19	4 g	(1 tsp of sugar)
Rice Krispies	2 g	
Shredded Wheat	0 added sugar	
Oatmeal	less than 1 gram	
Wheat Flakes	low sugar	

Most children and adults are satisfied with ¾-1 cup of cereal with some nonfat milk; a sliced banana, peach, or seasonal fruit; and a piece of whole-wheat toast with butter or peanut butter.

Fat.Fat.Fat.

Fat aids in the formation of cell structure, the transporting of molecules such as protein and certain fat-soluble vitamins to the cells, the transmission of nerve impulses, and the production of metabolic precursors.

There are certain fats, essential fatty acids, that can't be manufactured by the body. The most significant is linoleic, a polyunsaturated fat found primarily in vegetable oils. Its function includes aiding your blood's ability to clot, supplying padding for your organs, improving skin integrity, and aiding in hormone production. Too little fat intake is not a common problem for most people; however, if your fat intake makes up only 10% or less of a diet's daily calories, the body can't obtain adequate amounts of the essential fatty acids it needs.

Fat makes you feel satisfied. Fat is in meats, salad dressing, nuts, fast food, and a lot of snack foods like chips and dips. ***Fat has nine calories per gram, twice that of protein or carbohydrates,*** so watch your fat intake if you are overweight or if you have a family history of heart disease. Actually, everyone needs to be aware of the amount

Nutrient Basics: Protein, Carbohydrates, and Fats

of fat they eat. Even skinny people can have high cholesterol levels because of their fat intake.

So what do you need to know? Use fat sparingly. ***One teaspoon of fat is five grams. For females, if you keep your intake between 30-40 grams per day, you should be in a healthy range. Males usually have a higher caloric intake and, hence, a higher intake of fat (40-50 grams per day).*** If you're very active and need more calories to maintain your weight, you may need to consume 50-60 grams of fat in a day. ***Total fat intake should make up about 30% of your total calories for the day.***

**Daily Calorie Intake and Fat Grams
(Based on 30% of Calories from Fat)**

Calories	Fat Grams
1000	28
1200	30
1400	30
1600	33
1800	36
2000	40
2200	44
2400	46

There are different types of fat. ***Monosaturated fat is a good type of fat that may actually help to reduce your cholesterol level. These include olive, safflower, sunflower, peanut and canola oil.*** Polyunsaturated fats include corn, sunflower and soybean oil. Eat these in place of saturated fats. ***Saturated fats are often solid at room temperature—like the white fat on a steak or the leftover grease from your hamburger. Saturated fat can block your arteries and lead to heart disease. You'll find the highest levels of saturated fat in butter, ice cream, cheese, and meats.***

You've probably heard of trans fatty acids. These raise your cholesterol level. ***Watch for the word "hydrogenated."***

It's a saturated form of fat. You'll find it in many snack foods, like cookies and chips. Instead, use tub margarine or liquid margarine, and avoid white shortening.

Saturated fats, to eat less of:

Cheese
Palm oil
Coconut oil
Ice cream
Cream
Butter
Fatty meat

Is it easy to control the amount of fat we eat? Yes. Just consider the food groups and how much fat comes from each group.

AMOUNT OF FAT IN FOOD GROUPS

Fruit—almost none
Vegetables—none (except for the butter you add)
Bread—almost none, unless you buy the breads with lots of seeds
Milk—none if you use nonfat or skim
Meats—fish: very low, unless fried; chicken: low, unless fried; pork and lean hamburger (7% fat): low
Fat—depends upon how much of the following you eat: butter, oil, fatty meats, salad dressing, candy bars, ice cream, cheese

The choice is up to you. It's rare to find someone who doesn't eat enough fat, unless it happens to be a mom who is extremely paranoid that her family members are going to become overweight and makes major restrictions. Once again, *the important thing is to make gradual changes*. Your family will resist you if you become a "fat cop" and change everything overnight.

Since parents make the rules in most families, food MAY become a power issue. Here is the scenario: "I'll show you.

Nutrient Basics: Protein, Carbohydrates, and Fats

I'll sneak food when you aren't around. I will trade with my friends at school and eat their junk." You don't need food battles. If you start a healthy eating regimen when your children are young, or gradually make changes in their food choices, it's indeed easier to maintain the healthy eating mode. And, remember, it's never too late to make changes!

Think about the balance you do or do not have with the food choices you make for your family. Here are some assessment questions for you. If you find something you want to change or improve, write it down. Otherwise, praise yourself for your healthy choices.

1. We eat lean protein sources. ___yes ___no
Our plan for improvement: _____

2. We eat healthy carbohydrates, like fresh fruits and whole-grain cereals. ___yes ___no
Our plan for improvement: _____

3. We avoid fat from fast food and snacks and in our food preparation. ___yes ___no
Our plan for improvement: _____

Chapter Highlight:

Here's a quick recap!

Protein

1. Too much protein usually results in a high fat intake unless you're watching the fat content in your food choices.
2. A high-protein diet can be unhealthy for the kidneys and can affect the amount of calcium that your body absorbs.
3. It is pretty rare not to eat enough protein.

Carbohydrates

1. Carbohydrates are indeed your body's first choice for energy.
2. If you're eating a lot of simple carbohydrates, you may find yourself feeling fatigued and possibly bloated.
3. When you take in more carbohydrates than you burn, they will be converted to fat.

4. Think about it! Do you need two servings or five at your lunch? Are you going to be sitting at your desk or involved in basketball, tennis, or running this afternoon?

Fat

1. Fat is important. If you can pinch an inch, though, take a look at how much you're eating.
2. Switch from whole-milk cheese to low-fat cheese or from eating burgers four times a week to two times a week.
3. Be aware of where your fat is coming from (e.g., dairy, meats, snack foods, butter on your bread and potatoes, fried food).

What you eat is your choice. Food is not good or bad and does not make you a good or bad person. It does, however, have a big effect on your health!

Chapter Five

Green Tips

This chapter will review what you need to know if you are vegetarian or if you're thinking about becoming a vegetarian. I added this information after my experiences with young people who would declare they were vegetarian. Yes, they were vegetarian, but the quality of their diets was often weak. I found teenage girls who ate a few green salads during the day. Upon review, they were not compensating for eliminating all dairy nor did they pay attention to protein sources. Because they were often watching their weight, they didn't include legumes or nuts and actually had very low intakes of protein. My intention is to show you how to eat as a vegan, lacto-vegetarian, or lacto-ovo vegetarian and still have a healthy diet. In case you don't recall which foods are included or excluded, here is a quick review.

	Animal foods in diet	Foods not in diet
Vegan	none	all animal products
Lacto-vegetarian	dairy products	eggs, animal flesh
Lacto-ovo vegetarian	dairy products, eggs	any animal flesh

Vegetarian Eating Plans

Why even consider vegetarian eating? *According to the American Dietetic Association, scientific data suggests positive relationships between a vegetarian diet and reduced risk for several chronic degenerative diseases and conditions, including obesity, coronary artery disease, hypertension, diabetes mellitus, and some types of cancer.* Sounds good—right?

I ask patients to keep a three-day record and count how many servings they eat from different food groups and compare them to vegetarian guidelines, looking for any gaps or excesses. The three servings of milk, yogurt, or cheese will meet the calcium needs of most individuals. If you don't like dairy, you may want to supplement your calcium. Remember, you add to your bone density until your late 20s or early 30s. After that, it's a matter of daily replacement so that you don't end up with significant bone loss in your 50s and 60s. Since dairy is also high in protein, it doesn't take much to complete your protein needs, especially if cereals, whole grains, nuts, and seeds are added.

Food Guide for Vegetarian Meal Planning	
FATS, OILS, AND SWEETS—Use Sparingly candy, butter, margarine, salad dressing, cooking oil	
MILK, YOGURT, AND CHEESE GROUP **0-3 servings daily*** milk 1 cup yogurt 1 cup natural cheese 1 ½ oz *Vegetarians who choose not to use milk, yogurt, or cheese need to select other food sources rich in calcium.	**DRY BEANS, NUTS, SEEDS, EGGS, AND MEAT SUBSTITUTES GROUP** **2-3 servings daily** soy milk 1 cup cooked dry beans or peas ½ cup 1 egg or 2 egg whites nuts or seeds 2 tbsp tofu or tempeh ¼ cup peanut butter 2 tbsp
VEGETABLE GROUP **3-5 servings daily** cooked or chopped raw vegetables ½ cup raw leafy vegetables 1 cup	**FRUIT GROUP** **2-4 servings daily** juice ¾ cup dried fruit ¼ cup chopped raw fruit ½ cup canned fruit ½ cup 1 med fruit, such as banana, apple, or orange
BREAD, CEREAL, RICE, AND PASTA GROUP **6-11 servings daily** bread 1 slice ready-to-eat cereal 1 oz cooked cereal ½ cup cooked rice, pasta, or other grains ½ cup bagel ½	

Adapted from USDA Food Guide Pyramid

The vegan should be familiar with foods rich in calcium, B12, and Vitamin D. Most vitamin requirements are met by selecting from a variety of foods listed in the vegetarian pyramid.

If you are considering a vegetarian plan, it can be simple to eat a balanced, healthy diet. The addition of dry beans, nuts, seeds, eggs, and meat substitutes will easily meet your protein needs. One cup of most legumes, including black beans, lentils, or split peas, has 14-18 grams of protein. Most women only need about 46 grams of protein a day, and most men need around 56 grams of protein. As for your daily calcium needs, if you don't drink milk, select calcium-rich foods. Calcium needs are more easily met from a lacto-ovo vegetarian diet. Calcium is absorbed well from many plant foods. Vegan diets can provide adequate calcium if the diet regularly includes foods rich in calcium. Many vegetarian foods are now calcium-fortified and will help the vegetarian obtain adequate calcium.

Foods that Provide the Calcium Equivalent to a Glass of Milk

Almonds	6 oz
Beans, red	7 cups
Beans, white	2½ cups
Broccoli	2½ cups
Cabbage, green	3 cups
Cauliflower	4 cups
Mustard greens	1⅓ cups
Soy milk, unfortified	30 cups
Spinach	7¾ cups
Watercress	3½ cups
Fortified orange juice	1 cup

Vitamin B12 can be another concern for nonmeat eaters. The recommended daily intake is 1.8 to 2.4 mcg for teens and adults. B12 is used to develop blood cells. It is needed in order for your body to use folate, and B12 protects your nerve cells. Deficiency of B12 causes permanent nerve damage. Plant foods contain some vitamin B12 on their surface from soil residues, but this is not a reliable source of B12 for vegetarians. The B12 present in miso, spirulina, sea vegetables, and tempeh has been shown to be an inactive

B12 analog rather than the active vitamin. Dairy products and eggs contain vitamin B12, but research suggests that lacto-ovo vegetarians have low blood levels of vitamin B12. ***The use of fortified foods or supplementation is advised for vegetarians who avoid or limit animal foods.*** Many cereals, such as Total, are fortified with vitamins and include B12. Multivitamins are another option if you're not careful about your food selection.

Vitamin B-12 Micrograms per Serving

Ready-to-eat breakfast cereals, ¾ cup 1.5-6.0 mcg
Meat alternatives (made primarily of soy protein) 2.0--7.0 mcg
Fortified soymilk or other nondairy milks, 8 oz 0.2-5 mcg
Nutritional yeast (Red Star Vegetarian Support Formula, formerly T6635a), 1 tbsp 4.0 mcg

Another important vitamin to include is vitamin D, which is known to keep bones healthy. It works closely with calcium. ***Select vitamin D-fortified foods.*** Vegan diets may lack this nutrient because fortified cow's milk is its most common dietary source. However, vegan foods supplemented with vitamin D, such as soymilk and some cereals, are available. ***Sunlight exposure also affects vitamin D status.*** Sun exposure to the face, hands, and arms for 5 to 15 minutes per day is recommended. People who live in cloudy or smoggy areas may need increased exposure. Vitamin D supplements are recommended if exposure is inadequate. The elderly produce even less vitamin D and often have less sun exposure.

Vegetarian patients often ask me to design food plans for weight loss or maintenance.

The food servings for different calorie levels for vegetarians will vary. You may want to use a guide and write up a sample based on your personal food choices.

Food Servings for Vegetarians

Food Group/Servings	1200	1500	1800	2100	2400
Milk 90-100 cal/serving 8 g protein, 12 g carbohydrates	2	2	3	3	4
Fruit 60 cal/serving 15 g carbohydrates	4	7	8	8	9
Vegetables e.g., celery, lettuce, asparagus, mushrooms 10 g carbohydrates, 4 g protein 50 cal/cup	3	3	3	3	3
Grains e.g., rice, pasta, bread 15 g carbohydrates, 2 g protein 80 cal/serving	5	6	8	10	12
Protein meat substitutes 7-10 g protein 80 cal/serving	3	3	5	6	6

Fat	3	3	3	4	4
45 cal/serving—5 g fat or 1 tsp per serving					

The vegetables include all nonstarchy items like celery, radishes, mushrooms, tomatoes, artichokes, and asparagus. The grains include rice, pasta, and starchy legumes such as black beans, lima beans, or soy beans.

Many young people become vegetarian without knowledge of how to make the transition in a healthy way. The example reflects the application of a vegetarian diet for a college girl who wanted to lose weight.

FAMILY TIME

Susan was a freshman in college who had gained 20 pounds since she graduated from high school. She had recently decided she wanted to try a vegetarian diet. Her activity level was low. We designed a 1,200-calorie plan with the intention of building in extra calories as she increased her activity level. Many patients do better with serving ranges such as, "have three to four pieces of fruit a day or six to seven servings of bread" (depending on the activity level). Based on her food preferences, we came up with a food plan that looked like this:

Breakfast: 6 oz fat-free yogurt (1 milk)
½ cup cooked cereal or 1 slice whole-grain bread (1 grain); 1 tsp margarine or butter (1 fat); 1 small apple or 1 orange (1 fruit)
Lunch: 2 oz low-fat cheese (2 protein); 2 cups large green salad with red or green peppers and sliced tomato (2 vegetable); ½ cup legumes (1 grain); 2 tbsp seeds (2 fat); and 1 pear (one fruit)
Mid-Afternoon Snack: 15 grapes or 1 pear, or other fruit (1 fruit); ¼ cup nonfat cottage cheese (1 protein)

Dinner: 1 veggie burger (1 protein); 1 cup no-fat soy milk (1 milk); 1 whole-wheat bread with 1 tsp margarine (1 grain, 1 fat); ½ cup corn or peas (1 grain); 1 cup cauliflower, broccoli, or snow peas (1 vegetable)

Susan increased her activity level by finding time to walk 30 minutes daily. She lost six pounds the first month and reached her 20-pound goal in four months. She started her day with foods like oatmeal, fruit, and yogurt. She also kept one or two servings of fruit in her backpack, which made it easy to give up her mid-afternoon binges. The cafeteria wasn't fabulous, but there were always salad greens, legumes, and cheese available to add to her lunch.

At a follow-up visit at her next break, she was proud of the changes that she had been able to make. I reinforced that when she gets tired of the foods she's eating to take time to try new foods and improve the variety. We also reviewed how to fit protein bars into her food plan. For example, if the bar has 30 grams of carbohydrates, 10 grams of protein and five grams of fat, that's like having a sandwich with two slices of bread, one-plus ounces of protein, and a teaspoon of fat. I don't recommend replacing meals with protein bars—only in an emergency. I recommend not getting too far away from eating real food.

Whether you are an athlete in training, a woman sitting in an office, a professor in meetings and lecturing, or an executive who is on the go, you need to do some planning so that you aren't standing in front of the vending machine selecting a giant cookie and gummy bears for lunch.

Chapter Highlight: I've seen very few obese vegetarians in the past 20 years. If they were overweight, it was usually due to a high consumption of nuts and seeds. Consider this: ½ cup of soybean nuts is 390 calories, and ½ cup of almonds is 420. As long as you remember that they are not a "free" food, they're great in small quantities. Vegetarian diets are very filling due to their high fiber intake, and there are many tasty legumes and nuts that will give you good energy for hours.

Chapter Six

On the Go

Who doesn't want a lot of get-up-and-go? A complaint from many adults, especially women, is that they don't have enough energy. With the demands of a family, work, and many obligations, adults can't afford not to eat foods that will give them optimal energy levels. The frequent pattern is an afternoon binge at the candy machine, rather than a quick 20 minutes of exercise. Or no food until dinner, then . . . watch out! Better yet, look at exercise as your vitamin pill. It has *so* many positive side effects.

First, let's look at lifestyle causes of low energy levels: too little sleep, stress, skipping meals, too much sugar, and too little exercise. Fatigue can also be a sign of more serious conditions such as diabetes, heart disease, and cancer. Don't ignore your symptoms.

Recent research with cardiac and overweight patients, including adolescents, has shown that a low glycemic diet results in less hunger throughout the day. When you eat foods high in sugar and carbohydrates, the pancreas produces insulin that helps to transport the sugar in your blood into your cells, where glucose is converted to energy. Normally, the insulin receptors on the cells allow it to move glucose into the cells. In insulin resistance, the receptors don't recognize the insulin. As a result there's an increase in the amount of sugar and insulin circulating. The body produces the insulin but the cells are resistant to it. Hyperinsulin stimulates the appetite and increases fat storage in the abdomen. This has negative effects on your blood vessels.

The theory is that low-glycemic foods are less likely to cause increased insulin and blood-sugar levels and, hence, are less likely to stimulate your appetite. If you're trying to lose weight, you don't want to have your appetite continuously stimulated! Therefore, choose low-glycemic foods if you want to feel satisfied throughout the day.

You may also hear the term metabolic syndrome, known as Syndrome X, which is the same as insulin resistance. Characteristics of people with this common syndrome include: high triglycerides, low high-density lipoprotein (HDL), central obesity (you carry your fat in your midsection), elevated low-density lipoprotein (LDL), and hypertension. Your health professional may suspect that you have metabolic syndrome if you have some of these clinical indicators:

- Waist-hip ratio greater than 0.8 in women and greater than 0.95 in men
- Triglycerides greater than 150 mg/dl, HDL less than 40 mg/dl, and elevated LDL or total cholesterol
- Blood pressure greater than 140/90
- Acanthosis nigricans (skin that appears dark around the neck or under the arms)
- Elevated fasting blood glucose levels (greater than 126 mg/dl or a random blood glucose greater 200mg/dl)

If you know you have some of these characteristics, see your health professional regularly to prevent complications as you make diet and exercise changes. One study of patients who followed a low-glycemic diet for five weeks found positive changes in their serum lipids (refers to cholesterol and triglycerides) and improved postprandial (after-meal) blood-sugar levels and insulin profiles. In layman's terms, they reduced their risk for heart disease and diabetes. When patients select foods that result in a lower insulin response, they report greater satisfaction and control of their appetites.

Research also supports the use of a reduced-glycemic load diet for obese children. Rather than counting calories and fat grams, choosing low- and moderate-glycemic foods was more effective than a traditional low-fat, calorie-restricted diet in helping overweight children shed pounds and slow the progression of insulin resistance, a risk factor for diabetes.

This is not to suggest that you NEVER eat high-glycemic foods. You'll find you will feel better when you're eating foods that have less of an effect on your insulin level. Unlike many carbohydrates, protein foods do not tend to cause a high insulin response. Choose lean protein so that you don't end up with too much fat, too many calories, and little energy.

Gylcemic Index of Foods

GLYCEMIC INDEX OF FOODS		
Low Glycemic Foods	Moderate Glycemic Index	High Glycemic Index
Whole-wheat kernel bread Rye kernel bread All-Bran Cereal Fiber One Bran Cereal Unsweetened low-fat yogurt Apple Cherries Peach Pear Plum Lentils Red beans Baby lima beans Soy beans Spaghetti, protein enriched Tomatoes Asparagus, broccoli Brussels sprout Spinach, summer squash Tomato soup Peanuts, almonds, walnuts	Whole-wheat bread Cracked-wheat kernel bread Oat bran Kashi GOLEAN Oatmeal (slow cook) Corn Brown rice Bulgar Low-fat fruit yogurt Apple juice (unsweetened) Grapes Orange Dried apricots Canned pear in juice Canned chick peas Pinto beans Navy beans Macaroni (boiled 5 min) Green peas Sweet potato Canned lentil soup	Bagels Pita bread White bread Cheerios, Multi-Bran Chex Instant oatmeal, Puffed Kashi Shredded Wheat, Corn Flakes, Nutri-Grain, Cream of Wheat White rice Frozen yogurt Banana Mango Orange juice Raisins, watermelon, pineapple Canned baked beans Canned green beans Rice, pasta (brown) Spaghetti (boiled more than 20 min) Carrots, sweet corn, French fries, Winter squash Canned green peas, black beans Chips, crackers, cookies, honey

Here's an example of a sample daily menu:

Breakfast: All-Bran Cereal, nonfat milk, and an apple
Snack: nonfat yogurt and a peach
Lunch: salad with beans and lentils and 1 slice of whole-wheat bread
Snack: ¼ cup of walnuts or almonds and a cup of mixed fruit (peach, apple, pear)
Dinner: 4-6 oz of fish, a cup of protein-enriched spaghetti, salad, broccoli, and a cup of nonfat or low-fat milk

Another sample menu:

Breakfast: a cup of nonfat or low-fat yogurt with peaches
Snack: soy beans (edamame beans)
Lunch: tuna on salad greens or whole-wheat kernel bread, sliced tomatoes, and a cup of nonfat milk
Snack: ¼ cup walnuts or almonds, smoothie made with yogurt and seasonal fruit
Dinner: 4 oz lean protein of choice, ½ cup of baby lima beans, 1 cup of brussels sprouts, and a salad

The glycemic index guide has worked for many patients. I especially like it for the person who tells me they are hungry all the time. Trust me, it really works. You don't have to be rigid with it. Experiment with your food choices to see if you feel more satisfied throughout the day. Likewise, you can experiment with a day of eating high-glycemic foods and compare your energy level to a day of eating low-glycemic foods.

Here is an example of a low-energy teenager who changed his diet and experienced fantastic results.

FAMILY TIME

John was a 17-year-old overweight boy who complained of feeling sluggish. Although there was no family history of diabetes and his blood sugars were normal, we experimented with a low-glycemic food plan. He lost 15 pounds in about three months and reported renewed alertness. He also increased his activity level, adding to his mental and physical well-being! When you find a food plan that makes you feel good, you'll eat that way all the time, versus having low energy and wanting to sleep all day. When you find a food plan that makes you feel good, hopefully you'll try to eat that way all the time, just like John.

Chapter Highlight: Even though you may think this is another diet craze, please give this one a try. The improved energy level that some people have experienced is truly amazing.

Chapter Seven

Beat It!

Diet can affect cholesterol and triglyceride levels. Hyperlipidemia is the term your health professional may use to refer to an abnormal elevation of your blood (plasma) cholesterol and/or triglyceride levels. High levels of either may contribute to the formation of plaque in your arteries.

When my patients ask me for guidelines to reduce their cholesterol, I begin by suggesting they reduce their consumption of red meat to two to three times per week and lose weight if they are overweight. The majority of my patients with high cholesterol levels report they eat red meat on a daily basis. Even though diet isn't solely responsible for what shows up on your lipid panel, it does contribute.

Blood-cholesterol levels are affected by the cholesterol your liver produces, which you have no control over, and by your diet. High blood levels can also be suggestive of a triglyceride problem (see your doctor to sort out the cause). Most health professionals will give you at least a six-week trial period of diet and exercise before beginning medications to reduce your cholesterol level.

Cholesterol is in many of the foods we eat. The National Cholesterol Education Program recommends that you consume no more than 200 milligrams of cholesterol a day. If that doesn't reduce your cholesterol level, then reduce your daily intake to 100 milligrams per 1,000 calories. Therefore, if you think you consume 1,500 calories daily, it would equal 150 milligrams of cholesterol daily. The other fact to keep in mind is that your cholesterol level increases more from foods that are high in saturated fats. Saturated fats are usually solid at room temperature. If you see the word "hydrogenated" on a label, that's also a saturated fat.

Cholesterol in Certain Foods

	Milligrams
3 oz lean pork	67
3 oz lean beef	56
3 oz beef	90
3 oz light-meat chicken	85
3 oz flounder	58
3 oz salmon	74
3 oz crabmeat	76
3 oz lobster meat	72
1 large egg	218
1 oz cheddar cheese	30
1 cup cottage cheese, 1% fat	10
1 cup cottage cheese, 4% fat	34
1 cup skim milk	5
1 cup whole milk	33
1 tbsp butter	31

There are some new cholesterol-lowering margarines. They are made of plant sterols that actually compete with and stop cholesterol absorption in the body. Consumption of these sterols can reduce total cholesterol and LDL cholesterol. Benecol and Take Control are examples of cholesterol-lowering margarines. Three pats a day may improve your lipid levels.

Here's a summary of how to eat to reduce your cholesterol level. Review each category to see what you're already doing. For example, if you're already using Egg Beaters-great. If you haven't been including any fruit in your diet, set a goal now. If you have a fruit bowl in your kitchen, it will serve as a ready reminder to grab an apple or orange when you need a quick snack.

Food Guide to Reduce Cholesterol Level

Eat foods low in cholesterol	Avoid egg yolks. Use Egg Beaters, instead. Cut back on foods that come from animals. Try beans or soy foods instead of meats.
Eat more fiber and whole grains	Eat least five fruits and veggies each day. Eat whole-wheat breads and pastas, brown rice, and whole-grain cereals.
Eat foods low in saturated fat and trans fat	. Avoid: • high-fat meats, sauces, and gravies • full-fat milk and cheese • butter (use tub margarine) • deep-fried foods and snacks • store-bought baked goods • solid white shortening
Select vegetables seasoned with herbs or spices	Avoid: Sour cream, butter, or cheese. Ask for sauces on the side.

I find that many people are confused about the cholesterol terminology. Here's a brief review. Your doctor will probably measure your total blood cholesterol level. There are high-density fats (lipids) and low-density fats. ***The good ones are the high-density lipids (HDLs), and the bad ones that deposit cholesterol in your arteries are the low-density*** *lipids (LDLs).* It's good to know values of normal blood cholesterol and triglyceride levels.

Classification of Cholesterol Levels in High-Risk Children and Adolescents*

	Total Cholesterol mg/dl	LDL Cholesterol mg/dl
Acceptable	<170	<110
Borderline	170-199	110-129
High	> than or equal to 200	> than or equal to 130

Adapted from the National Cholesterol Education Program
*Children and adolescents from families with hypercholesterolemia or premature cardiovascular disease.

Adult Blood Cholesterol and Triglyceride Levels

Total Cholesterol

Desirable	<200
Borderline high	200-239
High	>240

LDL Cholesterol

Optimal	<100
Near optimal/above optimal	100-129
Borderline high	130-159
High	160-189
Very High	>190

Triglyceride

Normal	<150
Borderline high	150-199
High	200-499
Very high	>500

HDL Cholesterol

Low	<40
High	>60

Adapted from the National Cholesterol Education Program

Don't forget there are other risk factors besides high cholesterol that you need to be aware of to prevent heart disease, including: gender, family history of premature coronary heart disease, cigarette smoking, high blood pressure, low high-density lipid cholesterol concentration, diabetes mellitus, history of definite cerebrovascular or occlusive peripheral vascular disease, and severe obesity (greater than 30% overweight). As you can see, some things you just can't change.

Factors that appear to influence the HDL level are race, gender, body weight, smoking, alcohol intake, physical activity, hormones, and drugs. African-American males often have higher HDL levels than white males (cause is unknown); females have higher HDL levels than males; obesity is associated with lower HDL levels; cigarette smoking lowers HDL levels; moderate use of alcohol increases HDL levels; exercise increases HDL levels; estrogens increase HDL levels, and androgens lower them; and clofibrate, nicotinic acid, and heparin increase HDL levels, while zinc supplements lower them.

Low-density lipoproteins (LDL) are cholesterol-rich particles that transport cholesterol to peripheral tissues and possibly promote entrance of cholesterol into cells. The ratio of total cholesterol to HDL, indicating the balance between the cholesterol delivery and removal systems, may be more important than serum levels. An **ideal ratio** is under 3.5. A ratio lower than about 4.5 suggests that the risk for coronary heart disease is below average. A ratio higher than that offers a higher-than-average risk.

A note about **triglycerides:** they are the major lipid or fat in the body and in the diet. They add flavor and texture to foods. When blood levels are high, reducing total fat in the diet helps, as does reducing alcohol and carbohydrates (consumption of white sugar [and or] white flour). **Alcohol is strongly associated with high triglycerides.** High levels are seen in people who are diabetic, have kidney disease, or who are obese. Certain medications like thiazide diuretics, beta-adrenergic blockers, and estrogens may also increase triglyceride levels.

Individuals vary in their body's response to diet and exercise changes and their lipids. ***Research has proven that to make beneficial changes in LDL and HDL, adequate exercise is recommended of approximately one hour of endurance exercise per day, seven days per week.*** Physical impairments inhibit many people from reaching these goals, and medication therapy is often necessary.

Chapter Highlight: For a healthy heart, choose foods low in saturated fat, low in total fat, high in starch and fiber, low in cholesterol, and be physically active and maintain a healthy weight.

If you have children who eat fast food three to four times a week, regardless of their weight, you may want to check their cholesterol levels. Additionally, if there is a family history of hyperlipidemia, make this information known to your health-care provider. I have seen many children with total cholesterol levels above 220 mg/dl who were "normal weight."

Chapter Eight

Fiberlicious

One of my questions about body functions is, "Do you have any trouble with constipation?" Then, I like to throw in the comment that you know when you have enough fiber in your diet because your stool will float! "Ohh, really?" is the usual response.

First, why eat fiber?

- It helps keep you regular.
- It helps you fill up on less calories.
- It helps lower your blood cholesterol.
- It helps to reduce blood-sugar swings.
- It helps reduce the risk of diverticulosis.
- It helps in the treatment of diverticulosis.

All are important reasons. *A body needs about 25 to 35 grams per day.* I think the biggest misnomer is how much fiber is in salad greens. My sister was eating a big tostada the other day and commented on how the greens were such a good source of fiber. I hated to disappoint her, but half a head of lettuce has about .3 grams, and three stalks of celery has 1.5 grams of fiber.

As a rule of thumb, there is no fiber in meat or animal products. If you are on a high-protein diet, you may have a problem with your fiber intake! Fiber is in plant foods like fruits, vegetables, whole-grain breads and cereals, nuts, seeds, and beans. The white bread you're eating has .7 grams of fiber, compared with whole wheat that has 1.5 grams of fiber. Fresh vegetables are great for their vitamin and mineral content, and cooking doesn't destroy the fiber content.

Use this chart to figure out how much fiber you're eating in a day.

Fiber Content in Foods

Fruit (raw, canned, and frozen have about the same amount of fiber content, although the nutrients will vary)

	Total Fiber (in grams)
Raspberries (½ cup)	9.2
Blackberries (½ cup)	4.5
Pear (1 med)	4.0
Apple (1 med)	3.2
Kiwi (1 med)	3.4
Dates, pitted (4)	3.2
Blueberries (½ cup)	3.0
Orange (1 med)	2.8
Raisins (¼ cup)	2.5
Grapefruit (½ med)	1.1

Vegetables

Spinach (½ cup)	6.5
Squash, acorn (½ cup)	6.0
Peas (½ cup)	5.7
Corn (½ cup)	4.7
Broccoli (½ cup)	3.8
Sweet potato (1 small)	3.7
Baked potato (1 med)	2.6
Mashed potatoes (½ cup)	2.5
Eggplant (½ cup)	2.5
Brussels sprouts (½ cup)	2.3
Cabbage (½ cup, shredded)	2.1
Beans, green (½ cup)	2.1
Cucumber (1 med)	1.7
Carrot (1 med)	1.5
Asparagus (4 spears)	1.3
Peppers (½ cup)	1.0
Mushrooms (½ cup)	.8

Legumes

Kidney beans, cooked (1 cup)	19.4
Chick peas, cooked (1 cup)	18.2

Pinto beans, cooked (1 cup)	17.8
Split peas, cooked (1 cup)	10.2
White beans, cooked (1 cup)	15.8
Lentils, cooked (1 cup)	14.8
Lima beans, cooked (1 cup)	14.8

Breads and Cereals

Wheat bran (1 cup)	23.8
Cornmeal, dry (1 cup)	19.8
Wheat germ (3.5 oz)	9.5
All-Bran (⅓ cup)	8.6
All-Bran Bran Buds (⅓ cup)	7.8
Shredded Wheat (1 biscuit)	4.0
Wheatena cereal	4.5
Raisin Bran (½ cup)	4.0
Rice, brown, cooked (½ cup)	2.2
Bagel (1 med)	1.2
Bread, white	.7

Snacks

Brazil nuts (½ cup)	3.1
Almonds (13-15)	2.1
Popcorn (1 cup)	2.5
Sunflower seeds (¼ cup)	1.3

Fiber from oat bran, oatmeal, peas, beans, citrus fruits, strawberries, and apple pulp has been found to be effective in reducing cholesterol levels. Dietary fiber helps add bulk and increases water in the stool, helping to prevent constipation. It is important to increase your fiber intake gradually rather than suddenly to prevent increased gas or bloating. Drinking plenty of fluids as you increase your fiber intake will help prevent your stool from becoming hard. Fiber is also good for preventing and the treating hemorrhoids and diverticular disease. Fiber can make you feel full, which is a good thing if you are trying to lose weight.

Constipation is a common problem in children and a frequent cause of their stomachache complaints. **The** current recommendation for children's fiber intake is "age plus five." For children over two years, a safe range is "age plus five" up to "age plus 10" grams per day. For example, using this formula, a six-year-old should eat 11 to 16 grams of fiber per day.

Families are always surprised at how little fiber they eat. After looking at food lists and sources of fiber, they often find they're averaging 5 to 8 grams daily instead of the 25 to 35 recommended grams of fiber. When they find they are eating the appropriate or recommended amount of fiber, they are amazed at the filling effect of high-fiber foods.

Chapter Highlight: If you're eating plenty of fruits and vegetables, it's unlikely that you have a weight problem, a constipation problem, or that you are feeling hungry all day. Make fruits and vegetables available and eat them!

PART THREE

EATING ON THE GO

Chapter Nine

Planning Meals in Stride

This chapter will give you some easy, healthy meal plans for breakfast, lunch, snacks, and dinner. Pick and choose according to your taste buds!

One of the reasons a family may choose foods that are high in fat and sugar is that they are easy and initially satisfying. Check out your current food selections and see if your choices fall under "Healthy Choice" or "Room for Improvement."

Healthy Choice	*Room for Improvement*
BREAD SERVING	
Oatmeal or high-fiber cereal	Sweetened cereal
Whole-wheat bread	White bread
Small bagel	Large bagel (often equal to 4 bread servings)
	Scones
	Muffins
FRUIT SERVING	
Pears, bananas, oranges, or nectarines	Juices
MILK	
Nonfat milk, low-fat milk, or yogurt	Whole milk
PROTEIN	
Egg or egg whites	High-fat meats: sausage, bacon, or ham
Lean meat: turkey bacon	
Peanut butter (watch amounts if watching your weight)	

HEALTHY BREAKFAST FOODS TO GO

Apple and yogurt
Whole wheat bread and peanut butter
A baggy of Cheerios, ¼ cup raisins
Tangerine
Milk or yogurt
Small bagel with light cream cheese and raisins
Milk or yogurt
¼ cup nuts and raisins mixed in nonfat yogurt
Orange
Small container of cottage cheese with fruit and yogurt

It takes a little planning, but try not to skip a meal and set yourself up for overeating later. Make your grocery list weekly and put your favorite Healthy Choice basics on it.

LUNCHES

Many of my patients skip lunch. They claim they're too busy. That's not okay. Poor dietary habits lead to obesity and diabetes, which can be prevented simply by healthy eating and an activity plan to be on the right track. Here's a common scenario. Susan wakes up and downs a couple cups of coffee with half-and-half as she prepares her son's breakfast. She snacks on his leftovers and eats a couple of the cookies that she bought for his lunch. Then she's off to do her errands. She gets hungry while she's driving around, stops at a fast-food site for a burger and small fries, and she thinks she needs some sugar, so she also has a coke. She has so much to do that she isn't able to fit in her walk before her son gets out of school. She finds a few more cookies around the house when she returns home. By the end of the afternoon, Susan has had no fruit or vegetables and is wired on coffee and sugar. Daily repetition of fast-food burgers and sweets has left her 50 pounds overweight and out of shape. She has a sister with adult-onset diabetes, and her overweight mother developed diabetes at *age* 65. This is not a pretty picture, and she's not setting a good example for her son.

Planning Meals in Stride

How to Plan Ahead for a "Quick" Meal

I encourage families to plan "emergency" meals. This means they have healthy foods in their cupboards and can cook quick and easy healthy meals with very little thought or effort. What's in your cupboards that allows you to put together an easy but nutritious meal? Here are some healthy staples to have in your cupboards that would allow you to make a quick salad or sandwich.

Beans and Legumes: Find different beans or peas that you and your family enjoy and keep them in your cupboard, such as:

Garbanzo beans
Kidney beans
Pinto beans
Black beans
Peas
String beans
Pork and beans

Any of the beans can be mixed together for a good high-fiber, high-protein meal. Add a little olive oil, rice vinegar, and pepper, and you'll be surprised how filling and tasty beans can be.

Protein: Keep several sources of protein available, such as:
Hard-boiled eggs
Tuna, water-packed
Lean turkey or chicken
Feta or string cheese
Canned salmon or chicken
Edamame beans (keep these frozen and take out a handful for lunch)
Tofu cheese

Vegetables: Once again, you have lots of choices, fresh, frozen, or canned. Keep lots of fresh veggies on hand. Try eating at least two cups of veggies a day, whether eaten at lunch or dinner or split it up throughout the day with a few veggies at each meal. Keep fresh-cut veggies in the refrigerator to snack on. Without proper planning, it's easy to go a day or two without any vegetables.

Soups are another great option. Every family can use a slow cooker. Just add four to six vegetables and some broth. Soups are filling and can be frozen in individual or family-sized servings. You can also add tofu or lean meat for additional protein.

After-School Snacks

You and your children will eat what you have available. If you provide cookies, candy, ice cream, or Doritos, it will probably be everyone's first choice. However, if you have a fruit bowl in the kitchen, it's much easier to pick a piece of fruit to quench your late afternoon or pre-dinner hunger cravings.

Healthy Choices

Fruit
Fruit-flavored nonfat yogurt
Slice of whole-wheat bread with a slice of cheese or tablespoon of peanut butter
¼ cup of nuts
2 slices of cheese and whole-wheat crackers
1 tortilla and a slice of cheese
Veggies and dip

DINNER PLANS

When comparing eating out to planning dinner at home, realize you have a greater chance of healthy-sized portions of food when you dine together at home. Restaurants are fine if you're willing to scrutinize the menu. Moms often get burned out planning meals night after night. I recommend that when your children are 11 to 12 years old,

Planning Meals in Stride

make them responsible for planning dinner once a week. Some families also like to have a free night when everyone is on their own and can eat whatever they like that's available in the house. See how much fun this can be? And, you won't have battles if the right food choices are available.

Easy Choices for Dinners

> Lean protein—chicken turkey, pork tenderloin, scrambled egg or egg whites
> Soups—any but cream-based
> Homemade pizza—add your own tomato sauce, chopped vegetables, and lean meat or tofu
> Rice or baked potatoes with chopped vegetables and reduced-fat cheese
> Pasta

When you dine out, most restaurants have menus that support healthy food choices. If servings are large, share. Ask for your meat or fish grilled instead of breaded or fried. Ask for dressing on the side for your salad. Dip your fork into the dressing and drizzle it on your salad. Don't feel like you have to order an entrée. You may be satisfied with two appetizers or with sharing a salad and entrée.

Nothing is worse for the waist watcher than to order that fresh, tasty salad only to find it dripping in dressing. Most salad dressings are 70 to 100 calories per tablespoon. If you're not careful, that can mean an easy 500 calories from dressing alone. It takes practice to stop overeating. An important tip is to slow down, enjoy your food and work at stopping when you're "just satisfied." That's also another easy way to control caloric intake. Bag it up if there's too much food on your plate, and eat it the next day. I ask my patients if they prefer their excess to go on the waist or in the waste!

FAMILY TIME

The Smiths came to me for help with their eating choices. Dad had high cholesterol, Don, their 12-year-old son was

about 50 pounds overweight, and Mom skipped a lot of meals. They were concerned about their son's weight and Dad's medical problems. We reviewed their current eating styles, including the types of foods and amounts they ate, and their TV watching and activity level. Together we came up with a couple of changes they implemented.
1. They changed the types of food eaten at home, work, and school.
2. They selected cereals that were lower in sugar.
3. They began eating breakfast at home instead of stopping at a fast-food restaurant for ham-and-cheese sandwiches.
4. They limited TV watching to two shows a night maximum.
5. They began playing basketball or riding their bikes after school or dinner or played Frisbee in the park.

Goal for Parents: Be Good Role Models
1. Parents began eating with their son a minimum of three nights a week.
2. Parents expected son to go out and play before he watches TV after school.
3. Parents planned 30 minutes of activity most nights.

We talked about roles for parents and children. We decided that parents are responsible for the types of food in the house. (They agreed to stop bringing cookies and Pop-Tarts into the house.) Don wanted to be in charge of his physical activity. If he forgot, his Mom would remind him of no TV until he spent time exercising after school. The after-school activity became a good time to unwind and helped him avoid "stress eating." Mom was encouraged to spend time talking to Don after school discussing his day and encouraging him to share his activities at school and his feelings about things that happened that day. At first, he needed to be reminded to exercise. After a month, he began to take more responsibility. His mom bugged him less, and everyone seemed a lot happier. He had a few setbacks along the way when Dad would give in and take him out to eat before school, but that began to happen less often. No one felt like they were on diets, which helped alleviate stress for everyone.

Chapter Highlight: Plan your day. Don't give up and drive through the drive-thru because it's easier. The aforementioned list of quick and easy meals will help you get started. Add your favorite meals to the list so you'll have plenty of healthy choices.

Quick, Easy, and Healthy Meal Choices

Breakfast
1. Oatmeal, oat bran, or Cream of Wheat with skimmed milk, banana, or berries
2. Nonfat yogurt, sliced fruit sprinkled with oatmeal
3. Bowl of mixed fruit and slice of whole-wheat toast
4. Smoothie (blend skimmed milk, strawberries, and nonfat yogurt) and slice of toast or ½ bagel
5. Low-fat or nonfat cottage cheese and berries or other cut-up fruit
    *Use Benecol or Take Control margarine substitute if you have high cholesterol.

Snack Time
1. Apple, pear, orange, or banana
2. Carrots with fat-free ranch dip
3. Edamame beans
4. Nonfat yogurt with fruit
5. Baked sweet potato
6. Whole-wheat pita with hummus
7. Spicy tomato juice and whole-wheat crackers
8. Whole-wheat bread with peanut butter
9. Almonds, walnuts, or sunflower or pumpkin seeds (watch quantities)

Light but Filling Lunches
1. Lentil soup with whole-grain low-fat crackers, large salad, light dressing, and fruit
2. Vegetarian burger on half a bun with lettuce, tomato, and fruit
3. Tuna or chicken salad, one slice whole-wheat bread or ½ pita
4. Mixed beans (baked, black, kidney, garbanzo) with rice vinegar and fruit
5. Sliced sweet potato, nonfat yogurt, and fruit
6. Baked potato with Benecol, and large green salad with light ranch dressing
7. Bowl of nonfat yogurt, sliced fruit, and whole-grain bread and peanut butter
8. Chicken-breast sandwich and fruit

Dinner
1. Stir-fried vegetables with tofu, chicken, or shrimp and brown rice with a green salad
2. Vegetable soup (can be made in advance and frozen), green salad with light dressing, and fruit
3. Baked or grilled fish or chicken, baked potato, and steamed veggies or a salad
4. Scrambled eggs or Egg Beaters, whole-grain toast, and melon or other fruit
5. Steamed vegetables, protein-enriched spaghetti with tomato sauce, and fruit
6. ½ acorn squash filled with nonfat or low-fat cottage cheese, top with brown sugar or molasses

Chapter Ten

Fabulous and Healthy Recipes

I've saved "favorite" recipes for 20 years. This chapter includes my favorites. Hope you enjoy them as much as I do. Most have been analyzed for their protein, carbohydrates, and fats and fall within the "healthy guidelines." I used to always tell my guests which foods were "low-fat," but I don't announce this anymore as I noticed that friends who cook high-fat foods don't announce that their meal is "high-fat." Low-fat healthy eating is my style, and my friends and guests know that they'll be given healthy foods when they come to my house. Most are appreciative. Those who aren't I still hope to convert!

Recipes

Snacks, Appetizers, and Dips

Flavored Popcorn

Season with any of the following: grated parmesan cheese, garlic powder, cayenne pepper, or cinnamon.

Finger Jell-O

4 packages plain gelatin
3 packages sugar-free Jell-O
4 cups boiling water

Add water to gelatin and Jell-O powders and mix. Pour into pan and cool. Cut into squares and enjoy! Makes 16 servings.

Vegetable Dip

1 cup nonfat yogurt
1 cup fat-free sour cream

1 package Hidden Valley Ranch dry mix dressing
Serve with raw vegetables of your choice. Makes 16 servings.

Each serving provides:
20 calories
1.3 g protein
4 g carbohydrates
.02 g fat

Bean Dip

1 cup kidney, garbanzo, pinto, or black beans
1 tbsp chopped canned or fresh green chilies (optional)
½ tsp chili powder
1 tsp minced onion
pinch of cumin
1 tsp minced parsley
1 ½ tsp vinegar
Add to blender. Serve as spread or dip. Makes 8 servings.

Each serving provides:
27 calories
1.6 g protein
5 g carbohydrates
0.1 g fat

Artichoke Dip

1 cup nonfat cottage cheese
2 tbsp plain yogurt
¼ cup grated parmesan cheese
¼ tsp garlic powder and onion powder
14 oz can chopped artichoke hearts
Combine ingredients and blend until smooth.
Cover and chill. Serve with vegetables or whole-grain crackers. Makes 6 servings.

Each serving provides:
72 calories

5 g protein
4.9 g carbohydrates
4.4 g fat

Salmon Dip

1 large can of red sockeye salmon, drained
1 small onion, chopped
2 tsp dill
¼ tsp pepper
dash of salt
3 tbsp lemon juice

Mix ½ cup boiling water with 1 package gelatin. Dissolve. Add ½ cup light mayonnaise and mix with salmon. Add 1 small container of plain nonfat yogurt. Blend and refrigerate. Makes 16 servings.

Each serving provides:
123 calories
7.6 g protein
6.3 g carbohydrates
7.6 g fat

Spinach Squares

3 packages frozen chopped spinach
2 tbsp margarine (may use low-calorie)
¼ onion, chopped
4 oz mushrooms, chopped
6 eggs (use Egg Beaters)
1½ cup whole-wheat bread, cubed
1 tbsp Worcestershire sauce
2 cups nonfat cottage cheese
1 tbsp soy sauce
⅓ cup grated parmesan cheese

Cook and drain spinach. Sauté onions and mushrooms in margarine.
    Beat 6 eggs. Add bread, spinach, onions, mushrooms, and Worcestershire. Beat 2 eggs and add to cottage cheese with

soy sauce and mix. Combine mixtures and spread into pan and bake at 350° until knife comes out clean when inserted into center. For spicier squares, I add cayenne pepper or pepper sauce. You can also substitute 1 cup of cottage cheese with grated reduced-fat cheddar cheese. Makes 16 servings.

Each serving provides:
55 calories
5.1 g protein
3.7 g carbohydrates
2.1 g fat

Breakfast items

Yogurt Shake

½ cup plain or flavored yogurt
½ cup fresh or frozen fruit
¼ tsp vanilla
4 ice cubes
milk (optional)
Add a tsp of honey, if needed
Blend and serve. Makes 1 serving.

Each serving provides:
155 calories
8.6 g protein
28 g carbohydrates
.5 g fat

Banana Smoothie

1 med banana
1 cup skim milk
1 tsp vanilla extract
1 cup ice cubes
Blend and serve. Makes 1 serving.

Each serving provides:
194 calories

9.5 g protein
39 g carbohydrates
1 g fat

Sizzling Toast

1 slice toasted whole-wheat bread
1 teaspoon margarine
Spread with nonfat cottage cheese
Sprinkle with cinnamon and tiny amount of sugar
Broil 30 seconds and enjoy! Makes 1 serving.

Each serving provides:
151 calories
8.6 g protein
24 g carbohydrates
2.5 g fat

Fruit Broil

½ cup nonfat cottage cheese
¼ cup pineapple chunks
1 tbsp raisins
1 tbsp chopped walnuts or almonds
¼ cantaloupe
dash cinnamon
Mix cheese, pineapple, and raisins together. Add nuts. Scoop into melon and top with cinnamon. Broil 2-3 minutes until bubbly. Makes 2 servings.

Each serving provides:
110 calories
8 g protein
15 g carbohydrates
2.4 g fat

Apple-Raisin Muffins

1 cup whole-wheat flour
2 tsp baking powder

¼ tsp salt
1 tsp cinnamon
½ tsp allspice
1 cup bran
2 eggs
¼ canola or olive oil
4 tsp honey
1 tsp vanilla
1 cup skim milk or nonfat yogurt
1 cup chopped apple
½ cup raisins

Spray muffin tins. Sift flower, baking powder, salt, and spices. Stir in bran. Beat together with eggs, oil, honey, vanilla, and milk or yogurt. Stir in dry ingredients. Fold in apple and raisins. Bake at 375° for 20 minutes. Makes 15 muffins. (These may be frozen.)

Each muffin provides:
110 calories
3 g protein
16 g carbohydrates
4.5 g fat

Corn Bread Muffins

1 cup corn meal
½ cup nonfat yogurt
½ cup buttermilk
1 egg
1 cup whole-wheat flour
3 tbsp Butter Buds
2 tsp baking powder
½ tsp baking soda
1 tsp lemon zest
½ cup apple juice concentrate or other mixed fruit

Pour dry ingredients in bowl and mix. Add wet ingredients and stir. Bake at 350° for 20 minutes.

Makes 12 muffins.

Each muffin provides:
105 calories
3.2 g protein
17 g carbohydrates
2.9 g fat
18 mg cholesterol

Shirley's Bran Muffins

2 cups All-Bran Cereal
½ cup white flour
½ cup whole-wheat flour
1 ripe banana
1 tbsp baking powder
¼ tsp salt
1¼ cup nonfat milk
¼ cup Egg Beaters
¼ cup olive oil
¼ cup honey
1½ tsp cloves
½ tsp cinnamon
½ tsp ginger

Soak cereal in milk until soft. Add Egg Beaters, oil, and honey. Mix. Stir dry ingredients together, then add to wet mixture. Do not overstir. Adding walnuts and raisins are optional. Bake at 425° for 18 minutes or until lightly browned. Makes 12 muffins.

Each muffin provides:
144 calories
4 g protein
24 g carbohydrates
5 g fat

Cranberry Muffins

1⅓ cup whole-wheat flour
⅓ cup wheat germ
1 tbsp baking powder
¾ cup nonfat milk
⅓ cup honey
¼ cup egg substitute
2 tbsp oil
1 cup frozen cranberries, chopped

Stir liquid ingredients into dry ingredients. Coat muffin tins with spray. Bake at 375° for 25 minutes.

Each muffin provides:
112 calories
3.6 g protein
19.7 g carbohydrates
2.8 g fat

Fiberlicious Items (Vegetable Dishes)

Vegetarian Lasagna

1 cup cooked noodles
1 cup cooked frozen spinach
1 cup onion, chopped
1 tbsp oil
1 cup grated carrots
1 cup chopped mushrooms
½ cup tomato sauce
½ cup tomato paste (add a little water to this)
chopped olives (optional)
1 tsp oregano
1 cup nonfat cottage cheese
3.5 oz tofu
1 cup ricotta cheese (part-skim milk)
1 oz parmesan cheese, grated

Place noodles in a pot of boiling water for 8–10 minutes. Drain. Prepare spinach and drain. Sauté onion in oil until soft. Add carrots and mushrooms; cook until crisp-tender. Stir in tomato sauce, paste, olives, and oregano. Layer one half of each of the following: noodles, cottage cheese, ricotta, crumbled tofu, spinach, and sauce mixture. Repeat. Sprinkle with parmesan cheese. Bake for 30 minutes at 375°. Makes 8 servings.

You may experiment and add other vegetables or use different noodles, if you'd like.

Each serving provides:

270 calories per serving
20 g protein
28.7 g carbohydrates
9 g fat

Wild Rice
Always a hit!

1 cup wild rice
5½ cups chicken broth
1 cup yellow raisins
grated rind of one orange
¼ cup fresh mint
4 scallions, diced
¼ cup oil (optional)
⅓ cup fresh orange juice (may add more)
½ cup shelled pecan halves (optional)

Boil rice with broth. Mix the remainder of the ingredients together. May serve hot or cold. Dried cranberries are also good in place of raisins. Makes 12 servings.

Each serving provides:
118 calories
5.6 g protein
16 g carbohydrates
3.2 g fat

Summer Salad
Pretty and tasty!

10 cherry tomatoes, diced
½ pound fresh snow peas
½ cup sweet red pepper, diced
¼ cup green onions diced
10-12 basil leaves, sliced
10 oz package frozen corn, thawed
1 can drained black beans (optional)

Tomato Dressing
½ cup tomato sauce
2 tbsp golden raisins
2 tbsp white wine vinegar or rice vinegar
1 tbsp sliced green onions
3 fresh basil leaves
dash of salt
dash of red pepper

Combine ingredients and blend in mixer. Add to salad ingredients.
Blanch peas in boiling water for 30 seconds until crisp. Rinse with cold water until cool. Makes 6 servings.

Each serving provides:

120 calories
5.4 g protein
24 g carbohydrates
.7 g fat

Broccoli Souffle
5 cups broccoli florets
½ cup mushrooms, diced
1 cup diced onion

2 cups cooked rice
2 egg whites, whipped
1 cup low-fat cheddar cheese, grated
1 cup low-fat mozzarella cheese, grated
¾ cup nonfat milk
½ tsp garlic, powdered
¼ tsp white pepper
½ tsp thyme
2 tbsp low-sodium soy sauce

Sauté onions and mushrooms. Combine with broccoli, rice, cheese, and milk. Fold in egg whites, then bake in a casserole dish at 325° for 10-12 minutes or until mixture is firm. Makes 12 servings.

Each serving provides:
200 calories
16 g protein
24 g carbohydrates
4.9 g fat

Cynthia's Spinach Soufflé

10 oz package frozen, chopped spinach, thawed
16 oz nonfat cottage cheese
6 oz reduced fat cheddar cheese, grated
6 tsp flour
1 tbsp melted margarine
6 eggs (I use 3 egg yolks and 6 whites)
1 tbsp Worcestershire sauce
dash of cayenne pepper (if you like it spicy)

Add some nonfat milk if it needs more liquid. Beat ingredients together.
Pour into greased casserole dish and bake at 350° for 1 hour.
Sometimes I substitute 1 cup of chopped broccoli and 1 cup of chopped cauliflower for the spinach.
Makes 8 servings.

Each serving provides: (calculation based on use of 6 whole eggs)
192 calories
18 g protein
7.4 g carbohydrates
9.25 g fat

Lite French Fries

1 potato
1 egg white, unbeaten garlic powder, onion powder, or parmesan cheese

Adjust number of potatoes to your needs.
Bake at 425° for 25 minutes. Cut potato into strips and dip into egg white. Place on nonstick pan. Spray potatoes with vegetable spray. Sprinkle with powder or cheese. Broil fries for the last minute to make them crispier. Makes 1 serving.

Each serving provides:
130 calories
5 g protein
26 g carbohydrates
0.1 g fat

Salads and Dressings

Strawberry Poppy Seed Dressing

1 cup strawberries
½ banana
2 oz red wine vinegar
1 oz orange juice concentrate
1 tbsp poppy seeds

Puree banana and strawberries. Add vinegar, orange juice concentrate, and poppy seeds. Chill. Makes 8 servings.

Each serving provides:
25 calories

.5 g protein
4.9 g carbohydrates
0.5 g fat

Spinach and Strawberries with Honey Dressing

8-10 cups fresh spinach
2 tbsp balsamic vinegar
2 tbsp rice vinegar
1 tbsp honey
1 cup strawberries
1 tbsp sesame seeds, toasted
1 small red onion, sliced

Mix vinegars together. Add sliced strawberries, sesame seeds and sliced onion to spinach. Makes 8 servings.

Each serving provides:
35 calories
1.5 g protein
5.6 g carbohydrates
.7 g fat

Mixed Greens Recipe with Blue Cheese, Pears, and Pine Nuts
One of my favorites!

2 large ripe pears, diced (I also use granny smith apples as a substitute)
12 cups torn mixed greens (red leaf, curly endive, arugula, or Boston lettuce)
½ cup crumbled blue cheese (goat cheese or feta works also)
¼ cup pine nuts, toasted
salt to taste, black pepper
When ready to serve, scatter pears or apples over mixed greens. Sprinkle with cheese and pine nuts. May refrigerate up to 2 hours before eating. Makes 6 servings.

Each serving provides: (calculated with blue cheese)
119 calories
5.2 g protein
12 g carbohydrates
6.5 g fat

Honey Mustard Dressing

1 tbsp Dijon mustard
2 tbsp red wine vinegar
2 tbsp honey
4-5 tbsp oil or less (go as light as you desire on the oil)
1 tbsp water
salt (optional or to taste)
¾ tsp coarse black pepper
Shake together. Refrigerate until you serve. Makes 6 servings.

Each serving provides:
105 calories
.2 g protein
6 g carbohydrates
9.1 g fat

Rice Vinegar and Pineapple Dressing

1 cup pineapple juice
¼ cup rice vinegar
1 tsp lemon juice
¼ tsp dry mustard
One garlic clove
Optional ingredients to add: 2 tbsp celery hearts, chives, green onion, or red or green bell pepper
Mix ingredients until well blended. Add chopped vegetables last. Makes 8 servings.

Each serving provides:
21 calories
.1 g protein
4.7 g carbohydrates

0 g fat

Arugula Salad
Simple yet yummy!

1 bag of arugula greens (approximately 4-6 cups)
¼ cup grated fresh parmesan cheese or goat cheese
1 apple, pear, or 3 tbsp dried cranberries
1-2 tbsp toasted pine nuts

Dressing:
3 tbsp balsamic vinegar
1 tbsp orange juice concentrate
1 tbsp water
1 tsp Dijon mustard
1 tsp honey
1-2 tbsp olive oil

Makes 4 servings.

Each serving (with dressing) provides:
129 calories
3.8g protein
14 g carbohydrates
6.5g fat

Sheila's Balsamic Vinaigrette
4½ tbsp balsamic vinegar
½ cup fresh orange juice
4 tbsp squeezed lemon juice
4 tbsp olive oil
1 tbsp fresh or ½ tsp dried marjoram or oregano
pinch of cayenne pepper
pinch of ground black pepper
salt to taste

Combine in jar and shake well. Keeps for a week in the refrigerator. Makes 6 servings.

Each serving provides:
89 calories
.2 g protein
6.7 g carbohydrates
7 g fat

Sheila's Rosemary Vinaigrette Dressing

¼ cup oil
¼ cup chicken stock
1 tbsp white wine or rice wine vinegar
¼ cup fresh-squeezed lemon juice
2 tbsp fresh chopped or 1 tsp dried rosemary
1 tbsp Dijon mustard
½ tsp ground pepper
Combine in jar. Makes 1¼ cups. Keeps up to a week refrigerated. Good with arugula and radicchio greens.
Makes 6 servings.

Each serving provides:
68 calories
.4 g protein
1.2 g carbohydrates
7 g fat

PART FOUR

OVERWEIGHT? HOW TO LOSE IT!

Chapter Eleven

Ten Steps to Successful Weight Loss

This chapter contains content that I cover with my patients. I suggest that you highlight anything that is new for you. Weight management involves developing skills. You don't have to be perfect, but you've got to find a balance with your nutrition, exercise, and lifestyle in order to be healthy.

Is it useless to try to lose weight? No, no, no! Here are steps you can take to keep on target. I always remind patients that they've likely learned something from each and every program they've tried—you learn what works and what doesn't.

Step One: *Be honest* with yourself. Identify the contributors to why you're overweight. I use this scenario: If you were sitting in my office six months from now and were at your ideal weight, what habits do you think you would have changed to be successful? List them here.

Example: I would

- eat regular meals instead of going all day without eating
- limit my fast-food eating to once a week
- do some type of exercise four to five times a week for 30 minutes
- stop overeating
- not bring problem foods home
- not overeat when I go out to restaurants for dinner
- change my habits so that I don't gain 10 pounds when I go on vacation each year
- not overeat at holidays

- nurture myself without using food (friends, alone time, a good book, bubble bath)

Your turn. List all the bad habits you can think of that are keeping you fat.

1.
2.
3.
4.
5.

Now for the positive. List your strengths (good habits) that keep you from gaining more weight.

1.
2.
3.
4.
5.

Keep adding to your "strength" list as you develop positive habits.

Diets are hard to follow, and no one takes time to think about the underlying reasons they're overweight. Instead, they focus on the food they're going to have to give up. Negative thoughts aren't helpful. Losing weight is 95% mental. If you want to lose weight, you need to focus on the positive outcomes of losing weight in order to be successful.

Step Two: *One of the easiest ways to make changes is to pick one "target" habit and focus on changing that until it becomes a part of your life.* Don't pick the hardest one to begin with. When I lost 60 pounds, I started with a simple change of eating small regular meals instead of eating sporadically. I planned to have breakfast, a small snack if I was hungry, lunch, a mid-afternoon snack, and dinner. If I found myself going to the refrigerator at other times, I'd check myself and ask if I was really hungry. If not, I found something else to do. Many overeaters eat because they are bored, anxious, or depressed.

Buy a calendar and write your goal for the month on the top of the calendar. Then, each day, give yourself a check mark when you complete your goal.

Step Three: *Give yourself a safe food environment*, whether it's at home or at work. Here's a basic truth! If you offer healthy food to your family and yourself, and stock your cupboards and refrigerator/freezer with healthy choices, you're less likely to eat cookies. Even if you have a skinny spouse or thin children, they don't need to eat junk foods either.

Be a good role model. If this is a new step, take it slow or you may have a rebellion on your hands. Finish the sweetened cereals, and introduce less sugary cereals for yourself and family. At work, *bring* your lunch *from home* or think of what you can order when you go out to eat that has less fat and calories. Remember, it isn't the restaurant owner's goal for you to go away saying, "That was a thin serving!" Expect serving sizes that are at least twice the ideal size. Eat until you're satisfied and doggie-bag the rest for lunch or dinner tomorrow. At the market, buy only what's on your list. Nothing else!

Step Four: *Plan an exercise program.* Decide what you will do, when you will do it, and who you will do it with. Don't leave out ANY of these components. If you don't have a gym nearby, put on your walking shoes and walk. I look at exercise as my vitamin pill. If I don't do it, I have less energy. Moving my body makes me feel alert and strong.

Find something you like to do. When I started my personal weightloss program, I didn't have a gym and I wasn't a runner at the time. However, I did have Jane Fonda's exercise tape—not a video, just a little tape with music. She leads listeners through aerobic and strengthening exercises. I exercised to her tape five days a week. When I got tired of it, I changed my routine to an hour walk. When walking became too easy for me, I started jogging short distances. Eventually I began to run one mile, then three. Not everyone has the body for running or enjoys it like I do. Do what you love most.

Take your excuses and turn them into positive plans. I recorded my exercise on a calendar for about six years. I did this because my schedule varied. I was a student, a nurse, a teacher, et cetera. Each type of work brought a different schedule with it. Many times patients tell me that they don't have time. I challenge them to make the time. If it's important to you to have a healthy body, you can find the time. It may be that you need to walk 15 minutes at lunch and 15 minutes after dinner. Remember, the Surgeon General lists "not exercising" as a health risk just like smoking.

Step Five. *Determine your reasonable body weight.* You can use the Body Mass Index (BMI) to find a realistic range and healthy body weight, as we discussed in Chapter 2. Try to maintain a BMI of 24 or less. If you don't want to reach a goal of a BMI less than 25, remember that if you're overweight, even a loss of 10% of your weight will have positive health benefits!

Another simple formula often used to estimate weight is shown here:

Women

100 pounds for first five feet of height
5 pounds for each additional inch

Men

106 pounds for first five feet of height
6 pounds for each additional inch

Example: a 5'11" male should weigh approximately 172 pounds. (106 pounds for first 5 feet; 6 pounds x 11 inches = 66. 106 + 66 = 172)

Step Six: *Determine calorie needs to maintain and lose weight*

Current weight x 10 calories per pound (if inactive, overweight, frequent dieter)
Current weight x 13 calories per pound (active lifestyle)
Current weight x 15 calories per pound (for very active men and women who exercise five or more days per week for one hour or more)

Here's an example:

170-pound inactive sedentary woman
x 10 calories per pound
1,700 calories to maintain weight

Look at the difference in calories if this woman becomes active.
170
x13 calories per pound
2,210 calories to maintain weight

How much will you lose? If you want to lose one pound a week, cut back 500 calories a day.

Avoid eating fewer than 1,200 calories (for females) or 1,500 calories (for men) unless you are being medically supervised.

There are about 3,500 calories in a pound.

Example: The sedentary woman above required 1,700 calories to maintain her weight. 1,700 - 500

= 1,200 calories to lose one pound per week.

I don't recommend less than 1,200 calories because, if you're an active person, you're going to begin to feel too restricted in what you eat. I've included examples of food plans with different caloric levels. Your goal is to write a plan that will feel natural to you. You want a dietary plan that you can live with for life—not three days or two weeks.

Use the meal plan guide and plan a five-day menu. Here's an example using a 1,200-calorie daily guide:

Breakfast	Lunch	Dinner
Starch/bread 1	Starch/bread 1	Starch/bread 1
Meat 0	Meat 2	Meat 2
Fruit 1	Fruit 1	Fruit 1
Milk 1	Milk ½	Milk ½
Fat 0	Fat 1	Fat 1
	Vegetables 1 cup	Vegetables 1 cup
	Mid-afternoon snack 1 bread	

1,200 calories:	1,500 calories:	1,800 calories:
4 breads	7 breads/starches	8 breads/starches
5 meats	6 meats	6 meats
3 fruits	3 fruits	4 fruits
2 vegetables	2 vegetables	2 vegetables
2 fats	3 fats	4 fats
2 milk	2 milk	3 milk

Remember, these are not diets, but eating guides. They represent a healthy way of spreading out your energy (calories) for the day. Take a glance at the serving size and nutrients you receive from the various food groups.

Ten Steps to Successful Weight Loss

	Calories	Protein (g)	Carbohydrates (g)	Fat (g)
Milk	80	8	12	trace(tr)
(one cup nonfat)				
1 cup yogurt				
Meat, lean	80	7	tr	5
1 oz lean				
1 oz med fat	110	7		8
1 oz high fat	128	7		10
2/3 cup lentils	106	7.8	19	(tr)
Bread/starch	80	3	15	(tr)
1 slice				
1 tortilla				
pretzels ¾ oz				
popcorn 3 cups				
pasta ½ cup				
Fruit	60	tr	15	(tr)
½ banana				
½ cup juice				
Vegetable	25	2	5	(tr)
½ cup cooked				
1 cup raw				
Fat	45	tr	tr	5
1 tsp margarine				
1 tbsp nuts				
1 ⅛ avocado				

Step Seven: Problem-solve. Think about your past "problem foods," then brainstorm possible substitutions and a management plan. You don't have to promise you'll never eat a certain food again. When I was in college, my problem was strawberry drinks made with real ice cream.

Problem Food	Substitute or Sacrifice
1. Ice cream	Light ice cream
2. Macaroni and cheese	Use reduced-fat cheese
3. Candy	Limit to one or two small pieces daily
4. 3 glasses of wine/day	1 glass of wine per day
5. Chocolate	sugar-free cocoa or ½ candy bar or nonfat frozen yogurt

Step Eight. *Identify your high-risk situations and come up with a plan on how to avoid them,* or change your reaction to the situation. To prevent problematic eating, recognize your high-risk (red-flag) situations. List them below:

HIGH-RISK SITUATION	USUAL RESPONSE
1.	
2.	
3.	

Now, think about the occasion. What makes it a RED FLAG for you?

Brainstorm what your new response will be. Sometimes it helps to look at this diagram:

```
high-risk event ----- usual behavior ------ feeling

buffet meal ------ overeat --------- disgusted/fat
```

You have a choice of making a change in:

1. the high-risk event
2. your usual behavior
3. feeling

HOW?

The high-risk situation— avoid it if at all possible. If you're not ready to eat at buffets because you haven't developed the habit of stopping when you're just satisfied, then don't put yourself in an uncomfortable and vulnerable position! Otherwise, consider changing your behavior at buffets. For example, I use to plan ahead that I would taste a little bit of whatever I wanted, but my GOAL was to stop when I was JUST SATISFIED.

You'd be surprised how good it feels to leave a buffet with a comfortable stomach versus a bulging belly. Remember, just because you ate at a buffet doesn't entitle you to abuse your body by gorging it with excess food. Look at dining out as just another meal. That's really all it is! Your goal is to develop healthy eating habits in a variety of eating situations. If your PLAN doesn't work the first time, practice it again or try a new technique.

The last area to be conscious of is your feelings. Instead of dwelling on your guilt or disappointment, simply acknowledge that you need to try again. GO ON, FOCUS ON EATING HEALTHY. DON'T DWELL ON THE FACT THAT YOU SLIPPED UP!

Learn from the situation. Evaluate yourself after going through high-risk occasions. Are you noticing small changes indicating progress? If so, rejoice. If not, re-evaluate!

Holidays, birthdays, vacations, and transitions such as job changes, getting married, or moving, can all be stressful events that may result in changes in your weight. You aren't a failure; you just have to learn how to manage your eating in stressful situations. Create an action plan for managing each of your high-risk situations below.

HIGH-RISK EVENTS　　　　　**HOW I WILL MANAGE**

1.

2.

3.

4.

Step Nine. *Use positive self-talk daily.* What you think influences how you respond. If I tell everyone that I'm lazy, my failure to exercise every day isn't going to surprise anyone. However, if I say I'm getting fit, I will expect myself to perform activities that will lead to that condition. For example, if I say, "I am addicted to chocolate, and I expect to lose control every time I eat it, I wil probably lose control." Instead, if I say, "I like chocolate, and I choose to manage it by including it in my diet in small quantities," that's more positive and probable. Pat yourself on the back for the little positive things that you do every day that are just a little bit different than before. This shows you aren't just talking the talk but are JUST doing it, just like NIKE says. At the time I was overweight, I had heard the saying "nothing tastes as good as thin feels." Honestly, I found that to be true. All I had to do was recall those times in the bathroom when my sister and girlfriend would help me zip my pants because they were so tight!

Find someone to be your support person—perhaps your spouse or partner, a friend, daughter, parent(s), or support group. It helps to have someone to share with. If this isn't possible, consider beginning a journal of your efforts.

Step Ten. *Use food records or behavior records.* Use a chart and keep track of your food choices every day. It helps keep you focused. You can track how many fruits and veggies you're eating each day, or count your fat grams if fat intake is a problem. Establish clear goals and know what you expect of yourself. If you don't have a plan, trust me, nothing will happen!

Evaluate and re-evaluate. The process of losing weight involves learning and practicing new weight-management skills. Turn challenges into learning situations instead of looking at challenges hopelessly. Keep your weight in perspective. Remember, a 10-pound weight loss is going to make your heart very happy, but it won't happen overnight.

When you lose weight, get rid of your fat clothes or have them altered. Patients who have three sizes of clothing in their closets aren't expecting success.

Sometimes there's actually a feeling of disappointment when you've successfully achieved your goal weight. This is a normal reaction. I remember thinking "now what?" I had focused so much energy on my body and getting it in shape that I didn't think about what was to come when I achieved that goal. Actually, that's when the work begins, because your goal is to keep maintaining your weight, activity, and lifestyle. It's a way of life, a healthy life!

Chapter Highlight: Surround yourself with helpful information, from *SHAPE*, *Fitness*, or *Cooking Light* magazines. Find a mentor or partner who can help you achieve your goals. Take time to look at your goal each day and reflect on the good things you're doing for your body, your health, AND YOUR MIND!

APPENDIX A

WEB RESOURCES

The following are some of my favorite Web sites for nutrition information.

Aim for a Healthy Weight www.nhlbi.nih.gov/health/public/heart/obesity/lose_wt/index.htm

American Dietetic Association www.eatright.org

American Heart Association's Obesity Page www.heartinfo.org/mosamfat197.htm

Body Mass Index Information Site www.cdc.gov/nccdphp/dnpa/bmi/bmi-for-age.htm

Boston Obesity/Nutrition Research Center www.niddk.nih.gov/health/nutrit/research/boston.htm

Centers for Disease Control www.cdc.gov

Center for Food, Safety and Applied Nutrition www.foodsafety.gov

Centers for Obesity Research and Education www.uchsc.edu/core

Children Nutrition Research Center at Baylor College of Medicine www.bcm.tmc.edu/cnrc/

Guidelines on the Identification, Evaluation, and Treatment of Overweight and Obesity in Adults: The Evidence Report www.nhlbi.nih.gov/guidelines/obesity/ob_home.htm

Defeat Diabetes Foundation www.defeatdiabetes.org

Food and Nutrition Information Center www.nal.usda.gov/fnic/dga/

Harvard School of Public Health www.hsph.harvard.edu (search obesity)

Healthfinder www.healthfinder.gov (Healthfinder® is a gateway Web site linking consumers and professionals to over 6,000 health-information resources from the Federal Government)

Consumer Lab www.consumerLab.com (independent tests of herbals, vitamins and supplements)

International Food Information Council http://ific.org

International Association for the Study of Obesity www.iaso.org

Mayo Clinic for Healthy Eating and Healthy Weight www.mayoclinic.org

Medscape Women's Health www.womenshealth.medscape.com

National Cholesterol Education Program www.nhlbi.nih.gov/guidelines/cholesterol/index.htm

Nutrition Navigator www.navigator.tufts.edu/index.html

Patient Centered Assessment and Counseling for Exercise and Nutrition www.paceproject.org

Resource Center Weight-Management www.medstudents.medscape.com

Shape Up America! www.shapeup.org

Surgeon General's Call to Action on Obesity www.surgeongeneral.gov/topics/obesity/

U.S. Food and Drug Administration www.fda.gov

US Government nutrition information and materials www.nutrition.gov

US Government health directory www.healthfinder.gov

Weight Control Information Network http://win.niddk.nih.gov

APPENDIX B

HELPFUL WORKSHEETS (MAY BE COPIED)

Food and Exercise Record

DATE	BREAKFAST food amount	SNACK	LUNCH food amount	SNACK	DINNER food amount	DAILY TOTAL	MEAL PLAN	EXERCISE PLAN
						milk=	milk=	
						veg=	veg=	
						fruit=	fruit=	
						bread=	bread=	
						meat=	meat=	
						fat=	fat=	
						milk=	milk=	
						veg=	veg=	
						fruit=	fruit=	
						bread=	bread=	
						meat=	meat=	
						fat=	fat=	
						milk=	milk=	
						veg=	veg=	
						fruit=	fruit=	
						bread=	bread=	
						meat=	meat=	
						fat=	fat=	
						milk=	milk=	
						veg=	veg=	
						fruit=	fruit=	
						bread=	bread=	
						meat=	meat=	
						fat=	fat=	
						milk=	milk=	
						veg=	veg=	
						fruit=	fruit=	
						bread=	bread=	
						meat=	meat=	
						fat=	fat=	

GROCERY LIST

Breads/Grains

_____
_____
_____

Vegetables, fresh if possible

_____
_____
_____

Condiments/Spices/Herbs

_____
_____
_____

Cereals

_____
_____
_____

Fruit, fresh if possible

_____
_____
_____

Beverages/Water/Wine

_____
_____
_____

Pasta

_____
_____
_____

Juice, Vegetable/Fruit

_____
_____
_____

Margarines/Other Spreads

_____
_____
_____

Rice

_____
_____
_____

Lean Beef/Pork

_____
_____
_____

Miscellaneous

_____
_____
_____

Peanut Butter/Nuts

_____
_____
_____

Chicken/Turkey

_____
_____
_____

Beans/Legumes

_____
_____
_____

Cheese	Flour/Sugar/Oil	Canned Fish
_____	_____	_____
_____	_____	_____
_____	_____	_____

Salad Dressing	Yogurt, low-fat	Milk, low-fat, skim
_____	_____	_____
_____	_____	_____
_____	_____	_____

2 to 20 years: Boys
Body mass index-for-age percentiles

NAME _____

RECORD # _____

*To Calculate BMI: Weight (kg) ÷ Stature (cm) ÷ Stature (cm) x 10,000
or Weight (lb) ÷ Stature (in) ÷ Stature (in) x 703

Published May 30, 2000 (modified 10/16/00).
SOURCE: Developed by the National Center for Health Statistics in collaboration with
the National Center for Chronic Disease Prevention and Health Promotion (2000).
http://www.cdc.gov/growthcharts

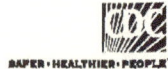

2 to 20 years: Girls
Body mass index-for-age percentiles

NAME _____
RECORD # _____

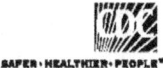

TARGET HABIT WORKSHEET

NAME: _____ DATE: _____

WEEKLY TARGET GOALS (be specific)

_____

_____

_____

_____

_____

ACCOMPLISHMENTS this week (fill in throughout the week)

_____

_____

_____

_____

_____

_____

_____

How I feel about my changes this week:

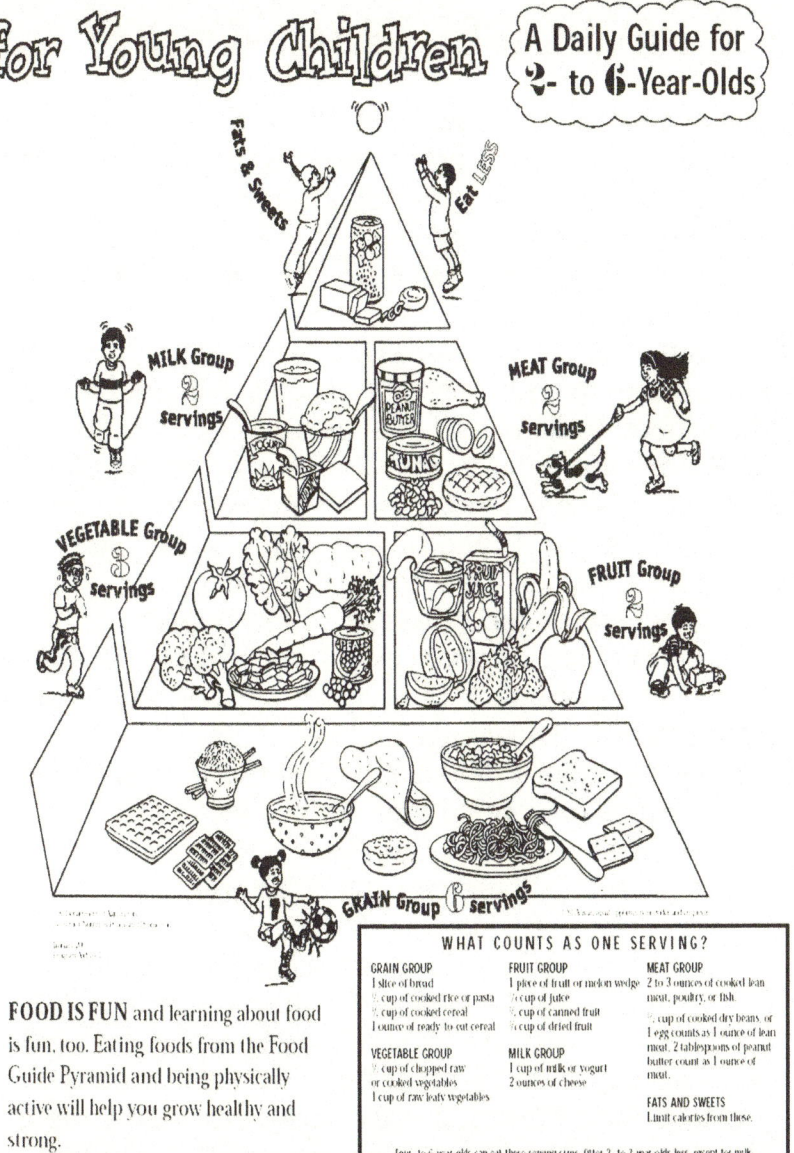

APPENDIX C

NEW LABEL TERMINOLOGY

Patients often ask how to sort out label reading. There are several new terms being used today. The following is information from www.cfsan.fda.govlabel.html.

DVs (Daily Values): a new dietary reference term that will appear on the food label. It is made up of two sets of references, DRVs and RDIs

DRVs (Daily Reference Values): a set of dietary references that applies to fat, saturated fat, cholesterol, carbohydrate, protein, fiber, sodium, and potassium

RDIs (Reference Daily Intakes): a set of dietary references based on the Recommended Dietary Allowances for essential vitamins and minerals and, in selected groups, protein. The name "RDI" replaces the term "U.S. RDA"

RDAs (Recommended Dietary Allowances): a set of estimated nutrient allowances established by the National Academy of Sciences. It is updated periodically to reflect current scientific knowledge

Whatever the calorie level, DRVs for the energy-producing nutrients are always calculated as follows:
- fat based on 30% of calories
- saturated fat based on 10% of calories
- carbohydrate based on 60% of calories
- protein based on 10% of calories (The DRV for protein applies only to adults and children over four. RDIs for protein for special groups have been established.)
- fiber based on 11.5 g of fiber per 1,000 calories

For labeling purposes, 2,000 calories has been established as the reference for calculating percent Daily Values. This level was chosen, in part, because many health experts say it approximates the maintenance calorie requirements of the group most often targeted for weight reduction and postmenopausal women.

For example, the Daily Value for fat, based on a 2,000-calorie diet, is 65 grams. A food that has 13 grams of fat per serving would state on the label that the "percent Daily Value" for fat is 20%.

It's important for people to know their *own* calorie needs, because DVs for the energy-producing nutrients—fat, carbohydrate, and protein—are based on recommended percentages of a total day's caloric intake.

Label Reading Summary

1. Serving size
2. Calories per serving
3. Calories from fat
4. Nutrients (You already have an idea of how much protein, fat, and cholesterol you should have each day. Too much fat, cholesterol, and sodium are not healthy.) Remember that the percent of Daily Value shown is based on someone who is consuming 2,000 calories.
5. Compare labels for the amount of nutrients the food provides, such as Vitamin A, Vitamin C, calcium, and iron.
6. Limit nutrients that have no percent Daily Value, like trans fat and sugars. Compare the labels of similar products and choose the food with the lowest amount.
7. A note about sugar: No daily reference value has been established because no recommendations have been made for the total amount of sugar to eat daily. Keep in mind, the sugar listed on the Nutrition Facts panel include naturally occurring sugars (like those in fruit and milk) as well as those added to a food or drink.

For more information about protein, calcium, and detailed label-reading guides, go to the Web site www.cfsan.fda.govlabel.html.

APPENDIX D

SELECTED REFERENCES

Bernstein, G. (2002). The diabetes epidemic: Keys to prevention, Guide to therapy. *Consultant*. May; 753-762.

Brosnan, C., Upchurch, S., Schreiner, B. (2001). Type 2 Diabetes in children and adolescents: An emerging disease. *Journal of Pediatric Health Care* Vol 15 (4), 187-193.

Blackburn, G., & Bevis, L. (2002). *The obesity epidemic: Prevention and treatment of the metabolic syndrome.* www.medscape.com/viewprogram/2015 (accessed Feb. 20, 2003).

Centers for Disease Control and Prevention. Basics about Overweight and Obesity. www.cdc.gov (accessed June 8, 2004).

Centers for Disease Control and Prevention. Body Mass Index for Adults. www.cdc.gov/nccdphp/dnpa/bmi/bmi-adult.htm (accessed February 8, 2004).

Center for Nutrition Policy and Promotion—Food Guide Pyramids. www.usda.gov/cnpp/pyramid.html (accessed June 15, 2004).

Clinical Guidelines on the Identification, Evaluation, and Treatment of Overweight and Obesity in Adults. Bethesda, Md.: US Department of Health and Human Services, Public Health Service, NIH, NHLBI, 1998. www.nhlbi.nih.gov (accessed April 8, 2004).

Insel,P., Turner,R. & Ross,D. (2003). Discovering nutrition. Sudberry, MA: Jones and Bartlett.

James, K. (2001) All in the family: Treating obesity in children and adolescents. *Advance for Nurse Practitioners*; 9: 26-33.

Mellin, L. (2003). SHAPEDOWN. (5th ed). San Anselmo, CA: Balboa Publishing.

Messina, V.K. & Burke, K.I. (1997). Vegetarian diets, position of American Dietetic Association. *Journal of American Dietetic Association,* 97, 1317-1321.

National Center for Health Statistics. (1999-2000). Prevalence of overweight and obesity among adults: United States, 1999-2000. www.cdc.gov/nchs/products/pubs/pubd/hestats/obese/obse99.htm (accessed October 3, 2003).

National Diabetes Education Program (NDEP) 1 Diabetes Way Bethesda, MD 20892-3600, 1-800-438-5383, www.ndep.nih.gov.

National Institute of Diabetes & Digestive & Kidney Diseases. (2003). Weight-control Information Network. www.niddk.nih.gov/health/nutrit/win.htm (accessed December 30, 2003).

Powell, K., Holt, S., & Brand-Miller, J. (2002). International table of glycemic index and glycemic load values: 2002. *American Journal of Clinical Nutrition*; 76: 5-56.

Third Report of the Expert Panel on Detection, Evaluation, and Treatment of High Blood Cholesterol in Adults (Adult Treatment Panel 111). National Cholesterol Education Program, National Heart, Lung and Blood Institute. National Institutes of Health; May 2001. NIH Publication No. 01-3670.

U.S. Department of Health and Human Services. (2001). Healthy People 2010: Understanding and Improving Health. Washington DC: US Government Printing Office.

INDEX

A
Alcohol 67

B
Breakfast 29, 36, 40, 41, 42, 43, 55, 61, 81, 86, 106

C
Calcium 52
Calories
  to lose weight 26
  to maintain weight 105
Carbohydrates 35, 39, 47, 107
Cereals 43, 71
Cholesterol
  Food Guide to Reduce Cholesterol 65
  food sources 51
Constipation 71

D
Dietary Guidelines for Americans 4
Dinner 30, 36, 40, 41, 42, 56, 61, 82, 106

F
Fatigue 57
Fats
  hydrogenated 45, 63
  polyunsaturated 44
  recommended amounts 72
  saturated 5, 45, 46, 63, 65, 68, 122
Fiber 43, 60, 69, 70, 71
Food Summary 21, 33

H
Heart disease 3, 4, 7, 9, 15, 16, 44, 45, 57, 58, 66, 67
High blood pressure 4, 15

N
Nuts 29, 95

O
Obesity and overweight classifications
  contributors 101

P
Protein
  food sources 51
  quick meals xii
  recommended amount 36

Q
Quick meal choices
  DINNER PLANS 78
  Lunches 82

R
Recipes
  Breakfast items 86
  Vegetable Dishes 90
Risk factors 15, 16

T
triglycerides xii, 15, 58, 67

V
Vitamin B-12 53
Vitamin D 51, 53

W
Weight loss
  Step Eight 108
  Step Five 104
  Step Four 103
  Step Nine 110
  Step One 101
  Step Six 105
  Step Ten 110
  Step Three 103
  Step Two 102

Made in the USA
Las Vegas, NV
03 May 2025

21656718R00083